Sedation, Suicide, and the Limits of Ethics

Sedation, Suicide, and the Limits of Ethics

James A. Dunson III

LEXINGTON BOOKS
Lanham • Boulder • New York • London

Published by Lexington Books
An imprint of The Rowman & Littlefield Publishing Group, Inc.
4501 Forbes Boulevard, Suite 200, Lanham, Maryland 20706
www.rowman.com

Unit A, Whitacre Mews, 26-34 Stannary Street, London SE11 4AB

British Library Cataloguing in Publication Information Available

Library of Congress Cataloging-in-Publication Data Available

ISBN 978-0-7391-9921-3 (cloth : alk. paper)
ISBN 978-0-7391-9922-0 (electronic)

∞™ The paper used in this publication meets the minimum requirements of American National Standard for Information Sciences Permanence of Paper for Printed Library Materials, ANSI/NISO Z39.48-1992.

Printed in the United States of America

For my parents, Sue and Jim, Jr.
who always support my academic endeavors
(whether or not they agree with my conclusions)

Contents

Introduction

In 2012, I decided to become a certified hospice volunteer. One day, I had a conversation with a patient with whom I played cards regularly when I volunteered. My patient was terminally ill and expected to live for only a few more months. On this day, he asked me whether it was wrong to pray to die. I was taken aback by the question. At that moment, I began to appreciate, insofar as I could, the strange situation in which he found himself: being completely cognizant of the fact that he was going to die in the very near future.

I regularly teach a college course in health ethics. The day after this conversation, I taught a section on end-of-life issues, specifically on the distinction between physician-assisted suicide (PAS) and continuous sedation until death (CSD). It occurred to me that the typical arguments on both sides of the debate over PAS would have seemed foreign to my patient. This was not because he lacked the technical expertise or mastery of jargon necessary for participating in the debate. Rather, the debate focused almost exclusively on the question of what policy we should adopt concerning end-of-life issues. But for my patient, the question of whether it was wrong to pray to die had nothing to do with policy formulation. He was contemplating what it means to live a good life and to hope for a good death.

I began to think that the standard debate over physician-assisted suicide was missing something important: an adequate appreciation for the *perspective of the patient* experiencing the dilemma. This observation is easy to dismiss at first glance. After all, the debate over PAS is not designed to give us an account of the subjective experience of the patient. This is especially true in the case of a utilitarian calculus that either supports or condemns this practice based on the greatest good for the greatest number. So it seems that a concern for the perspective of the patient might lead to an interesting discussion but that it is irrelevant in the context of the long-running debate over physician-assisted suicide.

However, I argue that our failure to focus on the specific dilemma in which my patient found himself has important policy implications. On my view, physician-assisted suicide should be recognized as a legally and morally permissible option for a very particular kind of patient: terminally ill with fewer than six months to live and capable of conscious consent. The permissibility of this option is not grounded in any of the traditional arguments that have been advanced in support of PAS. In particular, it is *not* based on a right to die. Instead, I argue that the legal and moral legitimacy of PAS in these circumstances derives from the well-established concept of informed consent. Making this option available to some patients would help to secure the kind of informed consent that is absolutely required in order to practice medicine.

Here is what I have in mind: When a PAS option is not available to patients who satisfy these specific criteria, then their options are limited in such a way that fails to guarantee sufficient informed consent. It is true that they have the right to refuse treatment and that they can be continuously sedated until death if the pain becomes otherwise unbearable. But in this process, they are compelled to live past the point of meaningful consent: Patients do not consent to terminal sedation because their capacity to do so has, by definition, already deteriorated. Further, as I show, most patients are not adequately informed about the effects of the superpharmaceuticals that we administer in the process of CSD. We operate under the assumption that patients would want to be rendered permanently unconscious if the alternative is suffering. Yet these patients are in this position because they were not presented with an alternative while they could still meaningfully consent. Giving these patients a PAS option months prior to continuously sedating them helps to ensure that they are both *informed* and *consenting* to the way in which they will inevitably die. In this way, having a PAS option is as important for those who decide not to exercise it as it is for those who do. To opt out of the PAS option is to actually consent to CSD. It is to genuinely choose, instead of passively receive, sedation at the end of life.

A narrowly circumscribed PAS option is important for safeguarding a respect for a patient's conscious experience of her end-of-life dilemma. At the heart of the need for informed consent is the idea that patients are not supposed to be passive recipients of medical expertise but rather active agents in their own care. Yet the prevailing norms concerning PAS and CSD reflect a clear concern for the patient's organism rather than her consciousness. She is permitted to refuse treatment and is promised superpharmaceuticals to treat her physiological pain. But she is not normally allowed to determine the timing of her death in a manner consistent with her values.

On my view, a PAS option is not an illicit request that competes with the right to refuse treatment. Rather, having this option *follows from* the refusal of treatment in just the same way as having access to morphine does. Pairing these two options (PAS and CSD) helps to protect a patient's ability to offer informed consent concerning her own demise. To the extent that a PAS option will help to promote informed consent for any particular patient, it should be recognized as a legally and morally permissible option.

Another effect of examining this end-of-life dilemma from the patient's perspective is that many of the traditional objections to PAS start to crumble. Take, for instance, the prohibition on the intentional killing of oneself and others. *From the patient's standpoint*, there does not seem to be much difference between physician-assisted suicide and continuous sedation until death. We have attempted to develop a clear consensus concerning how we define and diagnose death (e.g., irreversible cessation of all brain function, including the brain stem, or the complete and irreversible loss of cardiopulmonary function). But, judged from the patient's own experience, permanent unconsciousness seems like a sufficient condition for dying.

Moreover, the patient is put in this condition *intentionally* and not as a foreseen but regrettable side effect. In other words, the whole point of CSD is to ensure that the patient will not consciously experience pain. Likewise, the notion that a patient who exercises a PAS option is committing *suicide* starts to get murky. My hospice patient was not suicidal in any typical sense: He was considering different ways of dying that also occur at different times and in different phases. If his pain became unbearable, then he could expect to be provided with a sufficient amount of morphine. In the case of continuous sedation, his organism would outlive his consciousness. This complex series of events does not seem easily reduced to a simple claim about suicide, even though we use that term to describe this end-of-life option.

It is important to note here that I am *not* claiming we should stop the practice of continuous sedation. Given the current conceptual framework, this practice is absolutely necessary in order to relieve patient pain. Instead, I am challenging the ways in which we have framed these end-of-life issues. I am suggesting that a PAS option offered months earlier could help to ensure that a patient is both informed and consenting.

In order to explain and defend this series of claims, I have divided the book into three main parts. In chapters 1 and 2, I outline some problems with the standard debate over physician-assisted suicide. Then I present and explain my own alternative. Also, I give some reasons this alternative way of framing the problem has been obscured by the dominant policy paradigm.

In chapters 3 and 4, I show how focusing on the patient's experience of this end-of-life dilemma transforms some of the basic concepts we use to engage in the PAS debate. Here I specifically address the prohibition on the intentional killing of oneself and others. Finally, in chapters 5 and 6, I offer some observations about the future implications of my thesis. I address how my view combats some serious threats to the respect for a patient's conscious consent. Then I discuss the pedagogical implications of my view in an effort to determine how to teach future doctors, pharmacists, and other medical professionals about these end-of-life dilemmas.

This book can be read in two ways that are complementary but distinct. Stylistically, it is very different from other philosophical writings on end-of-life issues. There are numerous literary references and anecdotes and not a lot of complicated language. I wanted to adopt a style that reflects the existential dilemmas that I discuss, even while presenting a sustained defense of a policy claim. Someone interested in parsing a contribution to the field can treat this book as a typical work in medical ethics. Someone interested in contemplating patient dilemmas can regard it as a narrative about the state of medicine and patient care.

I am grateful for the many thoughtful comments and criticism from my friends and colleagues. Special thanks go out to my patient editor, Jana Hodges-Kluck; my mother, Sue Dunson, and brother, Joe Dunson; my partner, Sarah Meier; librarian extraordinaire Hannah White; friends Nathan Cook, Chris Edelman, and Paul Joseph; and all of my wonderful colleagues in the Department of Philosophy at Xavier University of Louisiana (Joe LeFevre, Thora Bayer, Robert Berman, Paul Schafer, Jason Berntsen, and Sarah Meier).

Part I

Chapter One

An Alternative Defense of Physician-Assisted Suicide

In his letter "On Old Age," the Stoic Seneca writes, "Let us cherish and love old age; for it is full of pleasure if one knows how to use it. Fruits are most welcome when almost over; youth is most charming at its close. . . . Each pleasure reserves to the end the greatest delights that it contains. *Life is most delightful when it is on the downward slope, but has not yet reached the abrupt decline*."[1]

Modern readers might be skeptical about such a claim. Perhaps it romanticizes old age. At the very least, it would seem foreign or even absurd to anyone whose culture glorifies youth. Seneca's own gruesome suicide, as recounted by Tacitus, only confirms these suspicions.[2] Ineptly killing oneself in response to Nero's accusation of treason is not likely to make Seneca the poster child for end-of-life issues.

Let us consider, however, whether the time before the "abrupt decline" is morally significant. This need not pertain to old age: Terminal illness does not discriminate. Suppose that someone, at whatever age, is diagnosed with terminal cancer. It is her life, and not yours or mine, that will be snuffed out imminently. It follows, then, that the way in which we circumscribe and frame her end-of-life options is both philosophically interesting and morally urgent.

In the twenty-first century, Seneca's "downward slope" is better described as a series of plateaus: Patients get better or worse in fits and starts, and medicine morphs into the management of chronic pain. Unfortunately, our ability to control symptoms and suffering far outstrips our capacity to cure disease. We can offer a patient radiation and chemotherapy in an effort to keep the progressing stomach cancer at bay, as well as superpharmaceuticals to tamp down the pain, but we cannot cure the cancer itself.

Under these conditions, Seneca's observation becomes even more poignant. The line between licit and illicit death is difficult to draw when terminally ill patients enjoy only momentary respites from accelerating down the downward slope. The topic of physician-assisted suicide (PAS) highlights this dilemma because it combines conscious consent (in the present) with the recognition of imminent death (within six months).[3]

This book offers an unconventional reflection on end-of-life issues, focusing especially on physician-assisted suicide and continuous sedation until death (CSD). As I discussed in the introduction, I defend the legal and moral permissibility of a PAS option for a very particular kind of patient. In order to do so, I challenge the current conceptual framework that drives this debate. Our preoccupation with policy formulation has obscured the perspective of the patient experiencing this dilemma. The outcome of exploring this perspective is either an intuitive appreciation for why it matters that she, and not you nor I, is the one forced to consciously confront her own mortality. Or, to press the policy implications, it is a recognition of our failure to achieve sufficient informed consent from patients at the end of life.

As explained in the introduction, my claim is that pairing a PAS option with the practice of continuous sedation helps to promote informed consent. Doctors and patients should have honest and informed conversations about the process of dying over the final six months. Patients should understand the effects of the superpharmaceuticals that get administered on the presumption that terminal sedation is preferable to suffering. Finally, they should have access to a PAS option in order to participate consensually in the manner and timing of their own demise. Patients who make an informed choice *not* to expedite the process will have accepted in an informed and meaningful fashion what is now simply done to them.

My argument does not rely on any of the standard defenses of physician-assisted suicide. I do not argue that a patient has a right to die. However, it should be both legally and morally permissible for her to self-administer a fatal dose of barbiturates, given the dilemma in which she finds herself. A patient need not have a constitutional or moral right to something in order for it to be a permissible option. For instance, there is no right to continuous sedation until death, but it is ethically permissible. My argument is that PAS should be, too, and in just the same way. PAS helps to safeguard informed consent, so it is at the very least a necessary evil for some patients. I argue that this way of framing the debate over physician-assisted suicide avoids the conceptual traps and pitfalls that often plague proponents of PAS.

A whole host of arguments has been traditionally advanced against physician-assisted suicide, and they can be roughly grouped into three distinct but overlapping categories: 1) those concerning the patient making the decision, 2) those concerning the doctor participating in the act, and 3) those concerning the society that has explicitly condoned such a choice by making it legally permissible.[4] On this standard view, 1) the patient does not have a right to die, 2) doctors who assist in death are transgressing the moral boundaries of medicine, and 3) the impact of legitimizing a PAS option could put society on a slippery slope to all sorts of moral atrocities.[5]

Proponents of physician-assisted suicide who accept this way of framing the debate take on some extraordinary argumentative burdens. They must 1) articulate a legal and/or moral right to die, 2) defend the idea of beneficent killing, or 3) promote the idea of a right to an enjoyable quality of life, even at the risk of sliding down a slippery slope. But as soon as one accepts the burden of proving the existence of a right to request death, this complicated issue turns into a general referendum on suicide. In contrast to the impeccable logic of CSD, suicide is obviously a hotly contested practice even outside of a clinical setting.

Once doctors are charged with participating in a patient's suicide, or even given the duty to do so, the right to die becomes especially implausible. The point of medicine is to heal or at least to remedy symptoms, not to kill. Doctors and patients are legally and ethically prohibited from intending and causing death. No one is responsible for cancer, but we are responsible for the choice to treat its symptoms until it causes death or to intend and cause the death ourselves. Daniel Callahan casts this distinction as the difference between physical causality and moral culpability.[6] On his view, assisted suicide and euthanasia are metaphysically distinct from continuous sedation until death. They are requests that issue from the self (moral culpability), instead of refusals that result in death from an underlying disease (physical causality).

As long as the discussion is framed in terms of refusing versus requesting, freedom *from* will always trump freedom *to*: A refusal always beats a request, and if the consequence of that refusal is intractable pain, then morphine and its pharmacological cousins are the inevitable remedy.[7] But *even if* proponents of PAS could contrive interesting arguments to support any of the above claims, it is hard to see how they could convince their critics. Rhetorically, if not philosophically, proponents of physician-assisted suicide have often lost the game before it was even played.

Imagine a terminally ill patient who appears to be completely lucid and free from any overpowering constraints. She is not yet experiencing the kind of intractable pain that might mitigate her consent. She has been diagnosed with six months to live and has made repeated requests for a fatal dose of barbiturates to self-administer. Does her lucidity show that she is functioning in a rational fashion, or does the fact that she is requesting PAS suggest the presence of a powerful constraint, such as undiagnosed depression, that had not been noticed?

A clear and concise statement of this problem is offered by Thomas Mappes and David DeGrazia: "It would beg the question to assume—in an effort to justify paternalistic interventions—that all decisions to end or risk life are irrational . . . and therefore nonautonomous. But perhaps in the case of those outcomes that are usually considered highly undesirable (e.g., death or severe injury) *it should be presumed that the individual's choice is irrational and therefore nonautonomous*."[8]

When the problem of patient consent gets reduced to question-begging claims about the possibility of rational requests, then we have no reason to take patient values seriously. Further, stipulating that death is intrinsically undesirable avoids the question of whether a particular patient is actually constrained or not. And it makes it difficult, if not impossible, to see what it would take to convince someone that the right to die is legitimate, once he has ruled it out in his very *definition* of patient autonomy.

The most clever defense of a right to die that I have seen illustrates the problem with debating this issue in the standard way. The Canadian Supreme Court was asked to consider whether denying a patient access to physician-assisted suicide ironically deprives her of a right to life. Before her death in 2012 from an infection associated with Lou Gehrig's disease, Gloria Taylor was a key plaintiff in the case *Carter v. Canada*. In his short article "And When I Die: The Pro-Life Case for Assisted Suicide," Wayne Sumner clearly explains Ms. Taylor's reasoning as follows:

> Taylor had a progressive neurodegenerative condition and wished to control the manner and time of her death, instead of letting her illness dictate her fate. She knew that, as her motor functions deteriorated, she would eventually be unable to bring about her own death. At that point, however, she might not be ready to die, judging that her life was still worth living. Allowing her to request assistance from a physician would therefore empower her to live beyond that point of personal incapacity, while still retaining control over her own death. Denying her that option would, conversely, force her to end her life while she still had the physical ability to do so. The law would deprive her of weeks or months in which she could still enjoy a life worth living; therefore, it violated her right to life.[9]

This counterintuitive argument suggests that access to physician-assisted suicide preserves, rather than violates, one's right to life. But notice what Ms. Taylor must concede in order to make such a claim. The argument only works if she admits that she would be *compelled* to end her own life before she is ready to do so. In addition to giving the unseemly impression of blackmailing the state, such an admission tacitly grants that the decision to die was forced and not free. The state, then, would be both the recipient of her threat and the indirect cause of her suicide. But even if this "pro-life" case for assisted suicide were philosophically plausible, it does not seem very rhetorically appealing.

Claims about new rights (like the right to die) give the impression of a profound discovery, as if we have found buried treasure where no one else has looked. But for this very reason, these claims also appear as uninvited guests at a dinner party organized by close friends: It is easy to ignore new rights claims that fail to engage with the basic presuppositions of the dominant view. Cultural norms and long-standing traditions provide a hefty counterweight to any defense of this supposed right. It is no coincidence that the Supreme Court referred to English common law to establish that suicide could not be a protected right in the United States.[10]

Even if all of those hurdles are overcome, those who defend a right to die would still have to deal with the many ways it could be regulated by the states. As we have seen with recent abortion regulations in Oklahoma and Texas, there are lots of clever strategies for restricting access to something deemed to be a right.[11] Strict regulation arguably makes the right itself de facto unreal. Two strategies for regulating a right to die immediately come to mind. A new controlled substances act could prohibit doctors from writing prescriptions for barbiturates; a right to die does not entail the right to one's preferred method of death. This might dissuade some patients from invoking their newly discovered right. Another strategy might be to lobby drug manufacturers to stop the shipment of drugs used in assisted suicide. We have already seen European drug manufacturers, backed by the executive arm of the European Union, refuse to ship sodium thiopental for use in lethal injections.[12]

Participants on both sides of the standard debate want to secure patient rights, protect the integrity of medicine,[13] and avoid any undue social harms. But whether a right to physician-assisted suicide would accomplish any of these things is the question. Both sides wish to promote patient dignity. But whether PAS preserves or violates this is the subject of massive disagreement, and it is unclear what would even count as a convincing argument on either side.[14]

Perhaps it is for these reasons that the debate has gone somewhat stale. The arguments on both sides are so well rehearsed that it sometimes seems like nothing new can be said. Edmund Pellegrino, the eminent bioethicist and critic of PAS, even titled a 2001 article "Physician-Assisted Suicide and Euthanasia: Rebuttals of Rebuttals—The Moral Prohibition Remains."[15] Unless one is interested in rebutting the rebuttals of rebuttals almost two decades later, one must find some other way to approach this subject.

***

The way out of this impasse is to refuse to allow opponents of PAS to completely control the terms of the debate, both with respect to its argumentative burdens and to the very language we use to discuss this morally complex issue.[16] This means not only giving up "right to die" arguments but also completely reshaping how we think of the right to refuse treatment.

In fact, the ultimate response to a PAS claim is not so much an argument as an outright dismissal. If true, it undermines the need for any discussion or debate at all. It has been advanced by distinguished bioethicists and codified by the Supreme Court. The idea is that a right to die is unnecessary because patients already have the right to refuse treatment and access to superpharmaceuticals to ease their pain. Palliative sedation is so effective at relieving pain that Justice O'Connor, in the famous 1997 case of *Vacco v. Quill*, argued that no additional constitutional right to die is even necessary.[17] Pellegrino, in his aforementioned 2001 article, made the same argument. In 2008, the American Medical Association approved sedation to the point of continuous and permanent unconsciousness in cases of intractable and otherwise untreatable pain.[18]

This view can be distilled down into two intuitive and basically irrefutable ideas: 1) A patient has the right to refuse treatment, as forced medication is a form of battery, and 2) the refusal of treatment requires palliative sedation because the patient will otherwise suffer immensely.[19] When the amount of sedatives administered are sufficient to cause a permanent loss of consciousness, palliative sedation becomes terminal sedation or the continuous sedation until death. The patient is kept unconscious until the body dies from the underlying disease. These two premises are virtually incontrovertible: To reject them is to condone 1) battery and 2) suffering. Paired together, they form the foundation of an appealing default position on this controversial topic. PAS claims, however well articulated, become so much hot air: Patients already have everything they need in order to die a painless death. This default position, so the story goes, is medically, legally, and ethically defensible. Doctors treat the symptoms of an underlying disease until they diagnose death. Patients exercise their rights (freedom *from* unwanted incursions) and gratefully accept the superpharmaceuticals that will alleviate their pain. Every step is legally and morally sanctioned: Doctors and patients both have recognizably good intentions, and neither is causing the death in any way.

Even those who have identified some salient moral objections to CSD admit that it is necessary. For instance, David Orentlicher skewers the Supreme Court's logic in the two main PAS cases, even comparing CSD to slow euthanasia.[20] But he admits that the connection between treatment refusal and sedation is so tight that they require one another: If a patient is permitted to refuse treatment without access to sufficient amounts of morphine, she will suffer. But if she is given the morphine drip without being permitted to refuse treatment, her rights will be violated, and she will essentially remain in a permanent vegetative state. So in a country where refusal of treatment is a basic negative right, patients must have access to superpharmaceuticals.

Having staked out the default position, all of the burdens now fall to proponents of PAS either to refute one of the two premises or to show why

PAS should be recognized as an additional right. I have suggested that neither strategy is philosophically nor rhetorically palatable. But suppose we examine this thorny end-of-life issue from the standpoint of the patient. This would involve reframing the debate from a third-person, policy-oriented viewpoint to a first-person perspective based on a very specific and personal dilemma.

The key question from this new point of view is how best to secure informed consent at the end of life. Here, the inexorable logic of CSD is self-defeating, as it does not guarantee a sufficient degree of informed consent. If, as critics freely admit, treatment refusal practically requires sedation, these two actions are still analytically distinct. In other words, one can imagine choosing one but not the other, even if (as Orentlicher concedes) it would cause harm to the patient. The patient freely consents to a refusal of treatment, but what about the continuous sedation of consciousness? Either this action requires free consent also, or it does not. If it does not require consent, then we might ask why, at this crucial end-of-life moment, informed consent is unnecessary. It was required at every moment until this final decision. On the other hand, if consent is required, then how is it secured?

We have reason to believe that it is not, in fact, sufficiently secured. In order for CSD to be legally and ethically permissible, it must be done when death is imminent.[21] Otherwise it would resemble euthanasia. But this means that the patient is already past the point of free consent. The pain has, by the very definition of CSD, already become intractable. So CSD remedies intractable pain when death is imminent, but it does so when consent can not be adequately secured. If consent is provided by a proxy in the family, we have reason to wonder why that outcome is preferable to prior patient consent. Arguing that proxy consent is required because patient consent is unobtainable begs the question: Is it unobtainable because the patient was required to live past the point of meaningful consent? I suppose that patients could claim in an advanced directive that they do not wish to undergo continuous sedation until death. But it is totally unreasonable to believe that this would be effective, especially when the document could simply be overridden once the patient is in the throes of unbearable pain.

Perhaps consent to CSD is implied when a patient refuses treatment. What, then, is the patient consenting to, and is that consent properly informed? In 2010, the Mayo Clinic published an informative guide to palliative sedation, in which providers are encouraged to inform patients that they will experience "a loss of social interaction."[22] This is the weakest possible formulation of what it means to be sedated, especially when it becomes continuous. My inability to communicate with my friends and family is not the primary effect. One step closer to an adequate description is the idea of "subjective death."[23] Patients should be cautioned that CSD will result in a permanent loss of consciousness. But to call this death subjective only makes sense from a third-person perspective. From a patient's standpoint, he will cease to exist.[24]

This formulation of continuous sedation is a yet another way of dismissing a patient's concerns: PAS is unnecessary because you already have access to CSD *and* continuous sedation causes merely subjective death.

The idea of subjective death also intimates that there is something we might call "objective death." This presumably lies squarely in the domain of science, so doctors are charged with diagnosing when the patient is objectively dead. This phrase also has an ethical connotation: Subjective death is neither scientifically real nor ethically relevant because the patient is not really (objectively) dead. The notion that subjective death is really "unconscious life"[25] is well established by the rules, policies, and procedures that we have adopted to deal with this question.

From at least as far back as the 1981 Uniform Determination of Death Act (hereafter UDDA), we have stipulated an exclusively organismic definition of death.[26] This uniform standard has been adopted, with slight modifications in some cases, by all fifty states. Its guiding principles have been codified in hospital ethics codes, and its logic has seeped into the very language we use when discussing end-of-life issues. The UDDA is a shining example of cooperation between medicine, law, and ethics: It was devised with input from the American Medical Association, the American Bar Association, and the President's Commission for the Study of Ethical Problems in Medicine and Biomedical and Behavioral Research. Their uniform standard is mercifully simple compared to the unwieldy title of the ethics commission itself: Patients are dead if and only if 1) there is irreversible loss of cardiopulmonary functions or 2) there is an irreversible loss of all brain function, including the brain stem.[27] This view confirms that CSD causes either a loss of social interaction or even subjective death, but it does not cause death in any objective sense.

Under normal conditions, the need for a uniform standard of death is obvious. If someone is catastrophically injured, doctors and families need some way of figuring out if that person is dead or alive. The last thing anyone wants in a time of crisis is a vague definition of death. If the need for a uniform definition is clear, then so is the requirement that it be physiological in nature: Whole brain death is diagnosable from a flat EEG.

However, in the context of CSD, we are faced with an interesting dilemma. If informed consent is required, as I think it must be, then the patient is 1) authorizing a doctor to deliberately induce an irreversible loss of consciousness and 2) consenting to the proposition that the organism that survives this loss of consciousness has, in a strange sense, superior moral standing. After all, it is not objective death (and therefore not killing) until the organism is dead by one of the two standards imposed by the UDDA. Consciousness may be irretrievably gone, but thankfully the brain stem is still functional.[28]

Even if these two outcomes were reasonable (and I do not think that they are), they would still be the product of a "choice" imposed on a patient 1) past the point of meaningful consent; 2) poorly articulated as the loss of social interaction or as merely subjective death; and 3) presented as an inevitable outcome.

Most damningly, this problem of informed consent is so intractable that conversations about patient values seldom even take place. A comprehensive 2014 study conducted by the American Medical Association identified some truly startling data on this problem. Among their many observations was the following: "Physicians do not routinely initiate end-of-life discussions until late in the course of illness. *In a large, population-based prospective cohort study of patients with metastatic lung and colorectal cancer, the first conversation about end-of-life care took place an average of 33 days before death.* Similarly, a large study of patients receiving dialysis found that 90% reported that their physicians had not discussed prognosis with them, despite an annual mortality rate of 22%."[29]

The so-called silver tsunami is fast approaching, even though our society is woefully lacking in geriatricians and other doctors who deal with end-of-life dilemmas.[30] Moreover, doctors who are already treating patients at the end of life rarely receive any training in conducting conversations about mortality.[31] Here, the authors of the American Medical Association study offer some provocative comments concerning the implications for informed consent: "Patients, in general, expect their physicians to initiate discussions about advance care planning and end-of-life preferences. *In this context, physician reluctance to broach these issues may prevent them from occurring at all, leaving physicians to make decisions about care without adequate information about patient's wishes.*"[32]

***

On my view, physician-assisted suicide helps to safeguard patient consent by making continuous sedation until death a free choice rather than an inevitable outcome. Having a PAS option does not mean having a right to die that goes beyond having the right to refuse treatment. Rather, it should be deemed permissible based on the fact that we *already* have the right to refuse treatment and access to superpharmaceuticals.

The relevant question, then, is not whether there is a right to die but instead what options should follow from my right to refuse treatment?

Here is how the logic of the argument goes: Concede the two incontrovertible premises involved in CSD (the right to refuse treatment and the need for palliative sedation). Also grant the general need for uniform end-of-life criteria. Then carve out an exception for patients who are terminally ill (fewer than six months to live) and sufficiently competent to have the kinds of conversations that usually do not take place.

These patients should have two options rather than one after giving notice that they will refuse treatment: They can either self-administer the dose and cause the death of their consciousness and organism at the same time, or they can opt for CSD instead. In either case, the patient as a person will cease to exist.[33] On my use of this term, personhood is inextricably connected to consciousness, but it need not be exclusively tied to moral status. In other words, all I mean by *personhood* is the capacity for conscious consent. Patients can decide for themselves whether their unconscious life is morally meaningful, and many will have good reasons for doing so. Suppose that a self-aware, terminally ill patient regards PAS as the ultimate evil. Suppose further that she views her own organism as the locus of moral value for her family and friends. There is nothing inconsistent with this view. But it does not rise to the level of a choice unless PAS is presented as an option.

If they choose CSD, then they explicitly endorse the medical, legal, and ethical consensus concerning death. They freely permit the doctor to effect the eradication of consciousness. Or maybe they simply believe that it is wrong to self-administer a fatal dose. On the other hand, if they choose PAS, then perhaps they believe that the irreversible loss of consciousness is a sufficient condition for death. Or perhaps they have some set of personal values that, were they to be properly informed about end-of-life practices, would lead to a strong PAS preference. Of course, we would still have to admit that a body with a functioning brain stem must be treated with some moral regard. We would not, for instance, begin an autopsy just yet. Notwithstanding this concession, the patient might be upset to learn that CSD compels her to consent to self-eradication, while stipulating that the real source of moral value is, in a sense, the organism. After all, it does not count as killing if only one's consciousness is irretrievably lost.

Physician-assisted suicide eliminates the gap between the eradication of one's consciousness and the death of one's organism. But while these perish simultaneously, it is likely that only the death of one's consciousness is morally significant for the PAS patient. So it is enough not to want to be compelled to care about the fate of one's brain stem, especially if it means living past the point of conscious awareness. Regardless of the outcome, the decision must be made only after doctors discuss the actual effects of both PAS and CSD rather than dismissing one as suicide and assuming the other as a medical, legal, and ethical default position.

In this way, recognizing PAS as a permissible end-of-life option helps us to honestly discuss and evaluate the difference between a person and an organism. This distinction is in fact *introduced* by CSD, which requires that the eradication of consciousness precede the death of the organism. So much for elegant end-of-life simplicity!

Patients who advocate for PAS are not choosing between life and death or between survival and suicide. They are stuck in a position where they are terminally ill and also sufficiently conscious of that fact. The standard rules and policies do not apply to them in the same way as the catastrophically injured patient who arrives in the ER already in a persistent vegetative state. Instead, they must have the option of taking the permanent eradication of consciousness seriously and regarding that as the only death that they will ever experience.

Further, they should have some say as to whether the different terms we use for sedation at the end of life are genuinely synonymous. Palliation is symptom relief: The goal is to ease a patient's pain once we have stopped trying to fight the disease. But continuous sedation until death is the intentional eradication of consciousness until the illness has caused the death of the organism.

Here is a different analogy: There is an obvious difference between administering morphine during a back surgery as opposed to giving morphine to induce a continuous state of unconsciousness. From a physiological perspective, the patient is unconsciously alive, and the doctor is alleviating the symptoms of the disease. But if CSD has been administered properly, the patient as a conscious entity has ceased to exist. This does not mean that there is a single moment in which we can be sure that the patient cannot feel pain. But once cessation of consciousness has been achieved, CSD can hardly be described as a *medical* option from the patient's perspective. The doctor continues to tend to the organism, but there is no longer a person benefitting.

So the excessive burdens that have been voluntarily assumed by proponents of a right to die should be reversed. Opponents of PAS should have the burden of explaining how CSD secures sufficient informed consent in the context of the most critical dilemma of one's life (i.e., when a patient is most starkly and absolutely an individual and when death comes for her and not for you or me).

One possible, or even likely, response will not work: dismissing the permanent loss of consciousness as a merely *subjective* problem. If, by way of contrast, the end of pain is an overriding and objective ethical concern, then CSD solves a problem that it created: A patient who chose PAS six months prior would avoid entirely the intractable pain that CSD is designed to remedy.

Also, since much of the case against physician-assisted suicide turns on the significance of patient and doctor intent, subjectivity matters *a lot* for those opposed to PAS. For this reason, it cannot be so readily dismissed. Patient intent determines, in part, whether an act counts as suicide. Doctor intent is relevant for assessing whether a patient has been killed or allowed to die from a disease. Further, the ethical support for the distinction between killing and letting die requires that any unintended harm done in the course of a good action be proportionate.[34] In other words, relieving pain is good, but I cannot deliberately kill the patient to end the pain. That would be disproportionate harm. But if the patient's perspective is merely subjective, then we have no way of weighing the end of suffering versus the permanent loss of consciousness. So we would not be able to satisfy the ethical criterion because we would have no way of knowing whether the putative harm was proportionate or not!

In fact, without a PAS option, continuous sedation until death becomes a Hobson's choice: The patient is offered the superpharmaceutical or nothing at all.[35] Let me rephrase: It is true that the patient could elect to have a lower dose of morphine, but she will likely suffer (perhaps unbearably) as a result. Since CSD takes place when the pain is otherwise intractable, suffering is built into the equation. If she had a previous choice to self-administer the fatal dose but elected not to do so, then the Hobson's choice becomes a genuine decision.

Let us use a hypothetical scenario to test our intuitions on patient choice. Suppose that PAS were the only option available to someone who decided to refuse treatment. Aside from any theoretical debate about suicide in general, we would have reason to object to the same Hobson's choice presented in the opposite way. Patients would feel compelled to self-administer the fatal dose in an attempt to avoid the intractable pain that awaits them. They would do so even if their values ran counter to such a decision. Now suppose that we legalize CSD to assuage patient concerns. Many patients would be genuinely relieved to have a second end-of-life option. Those who still prefer PAS would, for the very first time, genuinely choose it. Both options, then, are necessary.

Recall the double bind that makes CSD a necessary end-of-life option: If CSD is not an option, then a patient must choose between refusing treatment and accepting superpharmaceuticals. Since either option in isolation is terrible, it follows that CSD is required. But claiming that it is required is different from arguing that it is the *only* end-of-life option that should be available. And if having another option were to improve our ability to obtain informed consent, then it should be legally and morally permissible to offer it to dying patients.

My view asks what a patient needs in order to provide consent instead of establishing a new right that gets imposed upon a real dilemma. It grants a shared set of first principles (e.g., forced medication and intractable pain are both bad) instead of stipulating a new right that will strike critics as philosophically and psychological implausible. Aside from this basic difference between a right and a need, any rights claim is immediately generalizable, whereas patient needs are not. Even if there were a right to die, it would be almost impossible to limit this to conscious and consenting terminally ill patients. Why not let morbidly depressed patients or even depressed but otherwise healthy teenagers have access to fatal doses of barbiturates, too? They have a similar interest in individual autonomy and bodily integrity. Starting from the standpoint of a patient's needs means that the claims one makes are not similarly abstract and generalizable. In this way, it is possible to carve a meaningful PAS exception based on the dilemma faced by a conscious, terminally ill patient.

In the course of setting up my thesis for future chapters, I have rejected the standard arguments, burdens, and vocabulary of the PAS debate. I granted the two incontrovertible premises of a negative right to refuse treatment and a need for palliative sedation. I acknowledged that, under normal conditions, the medical, legal, and ethical default standard works just fine. My modest proposal concerns the permissibility of PAS as an end-of-life option that follows from the right to refuse treatment. A conscious, terminally ill patient is an ethical anomaly, and a PAS exception should be carved out in order to help safeguard informed consent at the end of life.

NOTES

1. Lucius Annaeus Seneca, *Moral Epistles*, trans. Richard M. Gummere, in the *Loeb Classical Library* 75 (Cambridge: Harvard University Press, 1917), vol. IV, epistle XII.
2. See Victoria Emma Pagán, ed., *A Companion to Tacitus* (Malden, MA: Wiley-Blackwell, 2012), 325.
3. Throughout my entire discussion of physician-assisted suicide, I assume the criteria outlined in Oregon's Death with Dignity Act (1994). This includes the requirement that the patient be diagnosed with six or fewer months to live. This legislation was approved by voters in 1994 and enacted in 1997. See Oregon Death with Dignity Act (1994) *Oregon Revised Statutes, 1996 Supplement*, 127.800-127.897.
4. The literature on the question of whether there is a right to die and how it should be evaluated is vast. For a clear discussion of the main issues, see Michael Cholbi, "No Last Resort: Pitting the Right to Die against the Right to Medical Self-Determination," *Journal of Ethics: An International Philosophical Review* 19 (2015): 143-157.
5. Supreme Court Justice Neil Gorsuch described the horrors that would be unleashed by the promotion of intentional killing, including "sadomasochist killings" and "mass suicide pacts" (153). See Neil Gorsuch, *The Future of Assisted Suicide and Euthanasia* (Princeton: Princeton University Press, 2009).
6. Daniel Callahan, "Killing and Allowing to Die," *Hastings Center Report* 19, special supplement (1989): 5-6. One way to understand Callahan's distinction is with reference to Hurricane Katrina in 2005. No one was responsible for the presence of a devastating hurricane (i.e., physical causality), but many people could be blamed for poor response times and failed levees (i.e., moral culpability). By analogy, cancer is a hurricane, and doctors are not responsible for deaths due to an underlying disease.
7. For a defense of treatment refusal as a sufficient substitute for assisted suicide based on the logic of refusing and requesting, see James L. Bernat, Bernard Gert, and R. Peter Mogielnicki, "Patient Refusal of Hydration and Nutrition: An Alternative to Physician-Assisted Suicide or Voluntary Active Euthanasia," *Archives of Internal Medicine* 153 (December 1993): 2723-28.
8. David DeGrazia and Thomas Mappes, *Biomedical Ethics* (New York: McGraw-Hill, 2011), 50.
9. Wayne Sumner, "And When I Die: The Pro-Life Case for Assisted Suicide," October 15, 2014, accessed December 4, 2015, http://thewalrus.ca/and-when-i-die/.

10. Chief Justice William H. Rehnquist used this exact logic when writing the opinion of the court in *Washington v. Glucksberg*, U.S. Supreme Court, 521 U.S. 702 (1997).

11. The Supreme Court invalidated some of these onerous restrictions in the case *Whole Woman's Health v. Hellerstedt*, decided June 27, 2016, accessed August 15, 2016, https://www.supremecourt.gov/opinions/15pdf/15-274_p8k0.pdf.

12. See Ian Steadman, "U.S. Prisons, Foiled by an EU Boycott, Are Turning to Untested Drugs in Executions," January 14, 2014, accessed March 25, 2015, http://www.newstatesman.com/future-proof/2014/01/us-prisons-foiled-eu-boycott-are-turning-untested-drugs-executions.

13. The relevant question is whether physician-assisted suicide is on the continuum of care or whether it is categorically different from treating patient pain.

14. An obvious instance of this disagreement is the Catholic Church's considerable opposition to the legalization of PAS in California. However, the concept of dignity need not have an explicitly religious connotation. It is easy to imagine someone making Kantian arguments against PAS based on the concept of the dignity of a person.

15. Edmund Pellegrino, "Physician-Assisted Suicide and Euthanasia: Rebuttals of Rebuttals—the Moral Prohibition Remains," *Journal of Medicine and Philosophy* 26 (2001): 93-100.

16. California's 2016 End of Life Option Act is a good example of these efforts to control the language we use to discuss PAS. It took effect on June 9, 2016 and was heavily influenced by the end-of-life advocacy of Brittany Maynard. Ms. Maynard was a terminally ill, twenty-nine-year-old woman who moved to Oregon to acquire a fatal dose of barbiturates. She published her own death date on Facebook. When the most populous state in America legalizes PAS as an arguably direct result of her actions, the consequences for the public are enormous. See Daniel E. Slotnik, "Brittany Maynard, 'Death with Dignity' Ally, Dies at 29," *New York Times*, November 3, 2014.

17. Justice Sandra Day O'Connor, concurring opinion in *Washington v. Glucksberg* and *Vacco v. Quill*, U.S. Supreme Court, 521 U.S. 702 (1997).

18. American Medical Association, *Code of Ethics*, Section 5.6, "Sedation to Unconsciousness in End-of-Life Care" (2016): 59, accessed March 3, 2015, http://www.ama-assn.org/ama/pub/physician-resources/medical-ethics/code-medical-ethics.page. This was based on a document with the same title, opinion 2.201, in 2008.

19. I understand that critics could argue that treatment refusal need not lead to immense suffering. However, no one would deny a patient access to morphine on the hope that she might die peacefully from starvation and dehydration. So the premise is still irrefutable as a general policy position, even if there could be outlier cases.

20. David Orentlicher, "The Supreme Court and Physician-Assisted Suicide: Rejecting Assisted Suicide but Embracing Euthanasia," *New England Journal of Medicine* 337 (1997): 1236-39. See also Margaret P. Battin, "Terminal Sedation: Pulling the Sheet over Our Eyes," *Hastings Center Report* 38, no.5 (2008): 27-30.

21. This is one of the criteria for sedation to unconsciousness referenced in the AMA Code of Ethics in note 18.

22. Molly Olsen, Keith Swetz, and Paul Mueller, "Ethical Decision Making with End-of-Life Care: Palliative Sedation and Withholding or Withdrawing Life-Sustaining Treatments," *Mayo Clinic Proceedings* 85 (2010): 951. The authors mention the loss of social interaction as a "foreseen likelihood." So not only is the loss of social interaction the weakest possible formulation of the effects of CSD, but also the authors do not even concede that it is more than a foreseen likelihood. In chapter 3, I discuss why we are not ethically permitted to assume that the negative outcomes of CSD are proportionate to its benefits.

23. This is sometimes how the permanent loss of consciousness is described by its critics. For a succinct account of some of these controversies, see Martin S. Pernick, "Back from the Grave: Recurring Controversies over Defining and Diagnosing Death in History," in Richard Zaner, ed., *Death: Beyond Whole-Brain Criteria* (Boston: Kluwer Academic, 1988).

24. Samuel Lipuma points this out in "Continuous Sedation until Death as Physician Assisted Suicide/Euthanasia: A Conceptual Analysis," *Journal of Medicine and Philosophy* 38 (2013): 190-204.

25. Josie Fisher makes this argument in "Re-examining Death: Against a Higher Brain Criterion," *Journal of Medical Ethics* 25 (1999): 473-76. Fisher concludes that we should have a conversation about the role of consciousness in making a life meaningful rather than redefining death itself. However, making a qualitative judgment about what makes life meaningful just invites a different kind of controversy. A debate over whether a life is worth living seems much more morally suspicious than debating how to define death in the first place. And even if we could agree on some necessary and sufficient criteria (which is highly unlikely), we might decide that "meaningless" lives are still worth living.

26. The Uniform Determination of Death Act was approved by the American Medical Association in 1980 and the American Bar Association in 1981.

27. The full text can be found on the Uniform Law Commission website, accessed October 20, 2015, http://www.uniformlaws.org/shared/docs/determination%20of%20death/udda80.pdf.

28. Here, as elsewhere, I am assuming that CSD *by definition* requires a permanent loss of consciousness. It is unconvincing to argue that the condition could be reversed, for then it would not count as CSD (i.e., it would not be continuous).

29. Rachelle E. Bernacki and Susan D. Block, "Communication about Serious Illness Care Goals: A Review and Synthesis of Best Practices," *JAMA Internal Medicine* 174, no.12 (December 2014): 1996, emphasis added.

30. See Stephen J. Bartels and John A. Naslund, "The Underside of the Silver Tsunami—Older Adults and Mental Health Care," *New England Journal of Medicine* 368 (2013): 493-96.

31. Bernacki and Block, "Communication about Serious Illness Care Goals," 1996.

32. Bernacki and Block, "Communication about Serious Illness Care Goals," 1996.

33. Here I am connecting the idea of personhood to consciousness. But as I explain, this claim relies only on a weak and *not* robust account of what personhood entails.

34. I have much more to say about this in my discussion of the doctrine of double effect in chapter 3.

35. A Hobson's choice is a "take it or leave it" offer that looks, at first glance, like a genuinely free choice.

Chapter Two

Ready to Die—An Existential Dilemma

A classic tale suitable for any book on end-of-life issues is the story of the death of Ivan Ilyich. Leo Tolstoy recounts the beautiful and unsettling coming to consciousness of a mid-level Russian bureaucrat. Ivan's previous confidence in his conventional success is undermined by an existential crisis that causes him to wonder whether his entire life was a lie. This crisis is occasioned by an injury sustained while hanging drapes in his home. A seemingly insignificant accident becomes the source of excruciating and ineradicable pain, resulting in his death several months later. The story ends with an epiphany and a presumed experience of the divine: "He sought his former accustomed fear of death and did not find it. 'Where is it? What death?' There was no fear because there was no death. In place of death there was light. 'So that's what it is!' he suddenly exclaimed aloud. 'What joy!'"[1]

This is a touching story of redemption, but my preferred end-of-life vignette comes from a different Russian existentialist. In his novel *The Idiot*, Fyodor Dostoevsky has the title character, Prince Myshkin, tell the story of a man facing execution. The three Yepanchin sisters listen with rapt attention. On his way to the firing squad, the condemned man has a sudden and terrifying realization: "What if I didn't have to die? What if I could get my life back—what an infinity it would be! And it would all be mine! Then I would make each minute into a whole lifetime, I would lose nothing, would account for each minute, waste nothing in vain!"[2]

Shortly after this realization, the condemned man's sentence is commuted. Here Prince Myshkin abruptly breaks off his account, and the confused sisters demand to learn the man's fate. Had he indeed lived according to the insight he was granted? The rince does not seem to grasp the urgency of their demand. He casually remarks, "Oh no, he told me himself—I'd already asked him about it—he didn't live like that at all, and wasted far too many minutes."[3]

This short story is buried in a big book, casually mentioned and then left behind. Unlike in Ivan's story, there is no great crescendo. Ivan's epiphany results in an experience of the divine, but the condemned man's epiphany culminates in an ordinary life. This combination of insight and banality makes the story in *The Idiot* less romantic and far more compelling. It reveals something about human nature and the crushing force of habit. Momentarily recognizing eternity in the present moment does not mean that one will actually live like a sage.

What makes the story from *The Idiot* even more captivating is that it mirrors Dostoevsky's own experience two decades prior. Having been sentenced to death for antigovernment agitation, Dostoevsky was lined up to be killed by a firing squad.[4] But like the character in the story, Dostoevsky's sentence was commuted at the last moment. He served out this sentence doing hard labor in a Siberian camp. It is not hard to imagine that Dostoevsky is describing his own attitude when confronted with his mortality. And perhaps he is also relating his own inability to live according to this crippling insight.

In the introduction and in chapter 1, I developed an argument in defense of making physician-assisted suicide a legally and morally permissible option for patients facing a special kind of dilemma: They are terminally ill, with fewer than six months to live, and they are sufficiently conscious of this. I claimed that a PAS option could help to safeguard informed consent in these cases and that there need not be a right to die in order to recognize this possibility. In fact, there is an enormous difference between deducing the legitimacy of PAS from a general right to die and showing inductively how a patient needs a PAS option given her current end-of-life dilemma.

In this chapter, I broaden the discussion in order to explore why this dilemma is seldom recognized as a problem of informed consent. I continue to argue that the concepts we employ in our attempt to formulate end-of-life policies end up obscuring the patient's perspective. Further, I argue that we are not sufficiently sensitive to the idea that a condition is *terminal* when we consider patient values. Finally, I claim that we defer far too often to the authority of scientific and ethical expertise concerning death and dying, even though these kinds of dilemmas in fact serve as a challenge to such authority.

If philosophy begins in wonder, then an individual contemplating her own mortality is surely one of the basic sources of intrigue. The contemplation of one's own nonexistence elicits all kinds of reactions, from denial of the inevitable to fear and trembling to gratitude to anticipation of spending eternity with God.[5] The astonishing diversity of funeral practices is a testament to this fact, from the traditional to the bizarre: the Irish wake, the New

Orleans second line, designated mourners in Mexico, and even Taiwanese funeral strippers. [6]

There is, in a sense, a way of denying one's own mortality: One can affirm an absolute faith in the divine and insist on the inevitability of an afterlife. But any religious person, no matter how devout, must at least consider the possibility of self-extinction, for this question resides in the realm of faith, not knowledge. Perhaps this is why even the most devout still mourn the death of a loved one. Regardless of our views on the possibility of an afterlife, we are faced with the certainty of our own extinction in this life *as we know it.* If the life that the devout are promised in the future would be different in kind from life as we know it now, then it would still count as a (now fortuitous) loss of self. So the point about self-extinction would still apply. On the other hand, if the afterlife is not different in kind from our present experience, then how much continuity is there, and how could this ever be known? No matter how strong one's faith is, the dilemma cannot be completely dissolved if one is naturally inquisitive. There will also be lingering questions, if not lingering doubt.

Seen from one perspective, death is completely commonplace and mundane. Until the Cartesian dream of solving the problem of death is finally realized, it is a necessary and inescapable part of the human condition. Yet seen from the inside, from a first- rather than third-person point of view, death is anything but banal. It marks the boundaries of an individual life, radically (perhaps even permanently) separating individuals from one another.

These two standpoints toward mortality might be described as the syllogistic approach and the existential approach. The classic syllogism proving Socrates's mortality is a testament to the universality and logical necessity of death: Socrates is a man; all men are mortal; therefore Socrates is mortal. But there seems to be an infinite gap between contemplating mortality as logically necessary and confronting my own mortality as a particular individual. What makes the story of the prisoner in *The Idiot* so fascinating is that it combines these two perspectives in a single character: from his momentary flash of insight to his return to ordinary life.

The logical proof proceeds with rational necessity, but the first-person point of view might better be characterized as absurd. If contemplating finitude in the abstract is categorically different from considering *my own* finitude, then these perspectives seem incommensurable and irreconcilable. In other words, we can think about death either from a first-person standpoint or a third-person perspective but not both simultaneously. Here we are left with a strange case of cognitive dissonance: In spite of the fact that we formulate rules, policies, and principles from the third-person perspective, we might also acknowledge that death is what individuates each of us absolutely.

There are many trivial and partially trivial ways in which we are our own individuals: One's favorite color and flavor of ice cream are individual preferences, but they do not mark us off as unique. After all, others can share our preferences, they can change over time, and (unless you are Ben or Jerry) no one would insist that these preferences make us who we are. Partially trivial differences might be something like taste in art and our political beliefs. Identifying oneself as a fan of Paul Gauguin or Ronald Reagan says more about us as individuals than our preference for rocky road. Claims about art and politics sometime even challenge others to search their own identity for commonalities or counterarguments.

If mortality is what ultimately individuates us, then perhaps our personal values regarding our own mortality should count as the least trivial, most absolute form of individuation. Suppose that one of us, but not both, will be here tomorrow: I but not you, or you but not me. Now we must face a dilemma: All end-of-life values are formed in the first- rather than third-person point of view. They are forged in the context of an individual life, possibly over the course of many years. Imagine a patient battling several bouts of cancer over the course of a decade, on a carousel of treatment, remission, and diagnosis. Whether these values are specified in an advance directive or just held privately, they are nonetheless personal in nature. You and I may both be mortal, but we are not Socrates, and we are not each other.

End-of-life issues are always existentially meaningful, but the stakes have been raised in the past century. If Ivan Ilyich were living in the twenty-first century, he would likely have more time to ponder his inevitable demise; there would be plenty of time for a deathbed conversion. As mentioned earlier, Seneca's downward slope has become a series of plateaus for patients fighting terminal illness. And thanks to incredible advances in public health and pharmaceutical development, we have dramatically increased life expectancy in general. We have ameliorated many of the harsh conditions that threatened human beings for centuries, even if the benefits have seldom been equitably enjoyed.[7]

As a result of this progress, the gap between the acute awareness of one's mortality and biological death itself has become a gaping chasm. Suppose that a relatively healthy ninety-year-old person were to decide that he has had enough of life. There is no evidence of depression (unless one believes that merely expressing that desire is sufficient proof). He fully understands that his life is coming to a close, and he is indescribably grateful for having lived a long and rich life. Still, he has outlived his family and friends, and he can no longer engage in the activities that used to make his life meaningful. Had he lived only one century earlier, all he would have to do is wait for pneumonia, the so-called "old man's friend," to kill him in a relatively peaceful fashion.[8] Now that we have battled this public health scourge, our hypothetical senior eventually becomes a reluctant centenarian.

Of course, none of this is to suggest that pneumonia should be left untreated or that the man in question should simply be allowed to die. My discussion of physician-assisted suicide has been carefully circumscribed to include only terminally ill patients who competently administer the fatal dose. But it is to suggest that there are interesting and unintended consequences of medical progress *for any particular patient.*

Progressive neurodegenerative disorders like ALS and Alzheimer's illustrate the gap between the awareness of one's mortality and one's inevitable demise. Suppose a patient is diagnosed with early-onset dementia, Alzheimer's type. The fact that we can identify this debilitating disease at its inception is remarkable. However, we have not made very much progress in curing Alzheimer's. The diagnosis is a death sentence delivered as a promissory note. In the case of ALS, we have developed eye-recognition software so that patients can communicate via computer even after much of their body has already shut down. But the same fate that befell Lou Gehrig in 1941 is now lying in wait for Steve Gleason.[9] Our sophisticated technology has undoubtedly improved the quality of life for people suffering from this terrible disorder. But it has also greatly increased the amount of time between diagnosis and death. The way in which particular patients respond to this fact is existentially interesting and morally significant. And the way in which we frame her end-of-life choices reveals a lot about the extent to which we think that her personal values are relevant.

***

We were told that no right to die is even necessary since the right to refuse treatment will inevitably include access to superpharmaceuticals. No patient needs to suffer once the pain has become intractable because she will be rendered unconscious. Yet CSD takes place a full six months after PAS becomes permissible. So it is a substitute for assisted suicide only if we believe that the patient's attitude toward those six months is not truly relevant. But on what grounds could we possibly say that?

It is true that both physician-assisted suicide and continuous sedation until death have an imminence criterion built in, but the meaning of the word *imminent* is completely different in the two cases. A patient cannot be rendered permanently unconscious unless the pain is otherwise untreatable and death fast approaches. A patient cannot avail himself of PAS unless his death is foreseeable within six months. If all we care about is ending physiological pain, then CSD might be a sufficient substitute for PAS. We would still have to set aside the concern that the inevitability of CSD creates the conditions under which the pain becomes intractable in the first place! But if a patient's consciousness of his impending demise is an important consideration, then the fact that PAS and CSD are separated by six months becomes morally relevant, too. It is unconvincing to argue that patient values are a crucial part of every medical decision made all the way to the end of life but that now the thing that matters most is alleviating physiological pain.

Eradicating pain is obviously going to be an overriding concern for a patient in the throes of suffering. But it cannot count as a reason for discrediting a patient's view on the significance of the six-month gap between PAS and CSD. We are compelled to care about the patient's first-person perspective, at least insofar as we must secure informed consent. This is a non-negotiable ethical consideration. So it will not suffice to say that pain is the only thing we need to really care about at the end of life. A patient is permitted to make that choice, but we cannot make it for her.

Take, for instance, some examples where we permit counterintuitive patient choices: A happy and healthy person can have a "Do Not Resuscitate" order drawn up at any time. Should some catastrophic event happen to her, we must honor her wishes, even if we think that her life is being irresponsibly cut short. Now imagine that she is a Jehovah's Witness who will need a blood transfusion in order to survive. The doctor's view is irrelevant: She can freely choose not to accept the blood, even if she will die as a result.

We are compelled to care about first-person attitudes and values, regardless of whether we agree with them. This should make us suspicious of the notion that CSD could serve as a sufficient substitute for PAS. For some concerned patients, CSD is not a substitute for PAS because it can come a full six months later. The two senses of the word *imminent* are not synonymous. If the gap between a patient's consciousness of her mortality and her biological death is morally meaningful, then we must be sensitive to her view on it.

Sometimes we are willing to admit this, but only in contexts *other than* PAS. Take, for example, the issue of whether chronically ill and catastrophically injured patients should be permitted to die by refusing treatment. The patients in question are not terminally ill; they include quadriplegics, brain stem stroke sufferers, patients with locked-in syndrome, and so on. Suppose that one of these patients wishes to refuse nutrition and hydration by forgoing a feeding tube. He also requests a sufficient amount of morphine so that he does not suffer. In cases like these, the impressive consensus forged by medicine, ethics, and the law in the Uniform Determination of Death Act starts to crumble. On one hand, no underlying disease is threatening to kill the patient. But on the other hand, the right to refuse treatment is supposed to be absolute: Forced medication is a form of battery.

The famous case of Elizabeth Bouvia became a flashpoint in the debate over the rights of patients with these conditions. In 1983, this twenty-six-year-old woman with cerebral palsy asked Riverside County Hospital to monitor her while she starved herself to death. She wished to refuse treatment and receive palliative sedation, but the hospital refused to comply. The medical staff did not want to participate in what they deemed a suicide.

Hospice administrators would not admit her because she was not dying from her condition.

Concerned parties thought it odd and even immoral to interpret treatment refusal as the deliberate decision to starve to death. Perhaps "treatment" should refer specifically to invasive procedures or poisonous chemotherapy. If food and water counts as treatment, then refusing it is not supposed to be the proximate cause of death. Further, it seemed strange to some that a patient could cause her own death by refusing questionable forms of treatment while simultaneously requesting morphine. If morphine is supposed to be medicine, then it, and not nutrition and hydration, most closely resembles treatment in this scenario.

In the case *Bouvia v. Superior Court*, the California Second District Court of Appeals upheld Ms. Bouvia's request to refuse treatment:

> All decisions permitting cessation of . . . life-support procedures to some degree hastened the arrival of death. In part, at least, this was permitted because the quality of life during the time remaining in those cases had been terribly diminished. In Elizabeth Bouvia's view the quality of her life has been diminished to the point of hopelessness, uselessness, unenjoyability, and frustration. She, as the patient, lying helplessly in bed, unable to care for herself, may consider her existence meaningless. She cannot be faulted for so concluding.[10]

The appeals court recognized the moral significance of the patient's own attitude toward her remaining years. Let us imagine that Ms. Bouvia might have lived another half-century if she had decided to endure her condition. The court deemed it relevant that she did not want to go on living in this way. They were willing to permit Ms. Bouvia to end her life a half-century early (based on this hypothetical timeline), as there is *no* imminence criterion for refusing treatment. However, critics of the court noticed the bleak and effusive rather than even-handed description of Ms. Bouvia's life. After all, she faced normal problems, too, like divorce and difficult job prospects. These critics claimed that the *Bouvia* case is about discrimination against people with disabilities, rather than a simple case of refusing treatment.[11]

When the U.S. Supreme Court rejected a constitutional right to die, the judges ironically shared some of the same concerns as the *critics* of the *Bouvia* verdict. In *Washington v. Glucksberg*, the court upheld a state ban on physician-assisted suicide (a decision that Washington voters reversed in 2008). The judges were especially concerned that vulnerable people might have their lives cut short if physician-assisted suicide were an option. Unscrupulous families might talk granny into permanently ending her pain. Well-meaning doctors might subtly coerce patients simply by presenting assisted suicide as an option. After all, death is not a rival form of treatment.

Chief Justice Rehnquist wrote, "The State's assisted-suicide ban reflects and reinforces its policy that the lives of terminally ill, disabled, and elderly people must be no less valued than the lives of the young and healthy, and that a seriously disabled person's suicidal impulses should be interpreted and treated the same way as anyone else's."[12]

This impassioned concern for the vulnerable might seem odd in light of the *Bouvia* verdict, where the California court was only too willing to agree with Ms. Bouvia's assessment of her condition. If one cares about the amount of time surrendered, then Ms. Bouvia would have only had to endure more than six months of her condition in order to outlive a hypothetical PAS candidate. This is not to diminish in any way her desire to die. But it is to point out a discrepancy in how we evaluate patient values.

The logic of the *Bouvia* verdict is impeccable in the context of the way the courts have interpreted the Equal Protection Clause: Equality does not mean treating everyone the same. Rather, it means treating like cases alike.[13] This requires that we determine what makes two distinct cases alike. We must carefully separate wheat from chaff, essence from accident. In treating like cases alike, Ms. Bouvia was counted as a member of a class of people who could invoke their right not to be assaulted through forced medication. Even though treatment refusal still requires "treatment" in the form of morphine (and despite the suspicious claim that food and water are medicine in this case), the legal and moral consensus says that switching off a machine is metaphysically distinct from allowing a patient to inject a fatal dose. So the California court could confidently agree with Ms. Bouvia's self-assessment since they were not technically condoning suicide.

All of this holds even though Ms. Bouvia clearly expressed her interest in committing suicide on several prior occasions.[14]

Ms. Bouvia was chronically but not terminally ill. Yet the California court endorsed her self-assessment because the distinction between refusing and requesting gave it license to do so. According to Rehnquist's logic, any similar statement about the suffering of a terminally ill patient who requests a fatal dose of barbiturates would count as discrimination against the vulnerable. This is true even though, in both cases, it is the patient's own *self*-assessment that is at issue. The terminally ill person making the request is not technically refusing treatment, so she is part of a different class of individuals. But this patient classification does not eliminate judgments about quality of life; it just makes us less able or willing to have an explicit discussion about it.

A patient's desire to die gets magically transformed into a legal right if (and only if) she can gain membership in the protected class. *This is true even if she is not terminally ill.* Instead, membership in the protected class is based on whether one is currently being treated for one's condition. There must be something to refuse in order to have one's wishes respected. On the other hand, membership in the unprotected group (those who "request" aid in dying) includes both patients who are terminally ill and those who are not. In rejecting a right to die, Rehnquist explicitly references patients who are terminally ill, disabled, and elderly. Yet one of these patients is not like the others!

Terminally ill patients are not choosing between life and death but between different kinds of death. For some of these patients, PAS and CSD are not substitutable methods because they care about more than just relief from unbearable pain. Those who refuse treatment have these desires taken seriously, even if they are not terminally ill. Patients who "request death" do not have these desires taken seriously, even if they are terminally ill.

***

If mortality is a source of nontrivial and even absolute individuation, then it is a serious ontological error to conflate two individuals who share the desire to die, though they may share nothing else in common. The fallacy of false equivalence points out the logical mistake of claiming that two views are equal, even though one side has substantially more evidence and arguments in support of it. In the case of end-of-life dilemmas, the superficial gloss given to these supposedly equal views is a shared desire to die. But the crucial differences between a terminal cancer patient requesting a fatal dose of barbiturates and a teenager contemplating suicide are thereby ignored. Both are regarded as instances of suicide, even though these two cases have virtually nothing in common. And the terminal cancer patient's request for barbiturates is seen as metaphysically distinct from another patient invoking her right to refuse chemotherapy, even though these patients may have the exact same diagnosis, prognosis, and hope for a peaceful death.

Both the court *and* its critics regarded Ms. Bouvia as a representative of other individuals in a common categorization. The debate was simply over which classification should trump. Did she represent a class of patients who wish to exercise their right to refuse treatment? Or was she a chronically disabled patient whose life was prejudicially demeaned by the court of appeals? In response to the disability activists who wished to protect her, Ms. Bouvia might have clarified that her desire to die was not an absolute statement about her disability or about the value of the lives of those who strive to live with chronic conditions. It is an obvious error to infer that one individual's desire to die means that all other individuals who supposedly share some basic similarity should have the same desire.

In these cases, we have located rationality in the *principle* rather than the *patient*: A patient's own self-assessment is irrelevant if our guiding principle (refusing versus requesting) categorizes her as a member of the unprotected class. On the other hand, Ms. Bouvia's attitude toward her remaining years was deemed by the appeals court to be a sufficient reason to let her die. It might be more accurate to say that the reasons for requesting PAS are not irrelevant so much as irrational: As soon as the debate over PAS becomes a referendum on suicide in general, some critics argue that such requests are inherently irrational.[15] Either we find some constraints and insist that they must override patient autonomy, or we assume at the outset that wanting an ordinarily undesirable outcome (e.g., death) suffices to show that the patient is acting irrationally. But in either case, there is no genuine and serious discussion of patient values.

A critic of PAS might be comfortable claiming that patient values become irrelevant as soon as a patient requests death. If such a request is legally and even metaphysically prohibited, then it can be ignored or even dismissed as irrational. However, there is no avoiding the question of whether a medical intervention would be a form of weak or strong paternalism. Since this question can only be answered by investigating possible constraints on a patient's ability to consent, PAS requests cannot simply be ignored. In other words, even if we want to dismiss the PAS request as irrational, we must still investigate the extent to which the patient is constrained. Otherwise we would not know how much intervention in her choices would be justifiable. And if it turned out that our policies governing CSD and PAS were strongly paternalistic, then we would have reason to evaluate whether they were justifiable at all.

The innumerable debates on paternalism are only superficially about the moral harm caused or averted by such interventions. Paternalism is philosophically interesting because it challenges us to carve up the world ontologically: Where does an individual patient's autonomy (and even identity) begin and end? Weak paternalism is the widely accepted idea that doctors and family members can intervene to restore autonomy when it is clearly constrained by a lack of understanding and informed consent, lack of intention, or the presence of internal or external constraints.

Terrence Ackerman, for instance, argues against the pernicious assumption that respect for autonomy entails nonintervention in patient choices. He reminds us of the transformative effects of illness, such that the very identity of the patient can be at least temporarily altered.[16] Under these conditions, respect for patient autonomy requires intervening to restore what has been lost. Strong paternalism, on the contrary, is the widely deplored notion that an autonomous and unconstrained adult should still have decisions made for her.

The difference between weak and strong paternalism is not simply about the moral harm imposed or prevented. The deeper difference is how we understand the very individuality and identity of the patient. In cases of weak paternalistic interventions, the patient is not herself, as she is constrained in various ways. In strong paternalism, the patient is an unconstrained, autonomous individual with her self-identity preserved. This is why one form of paternalism is morally permitted or even praised, while the other is condemned. From an outside perspective, the very same action can be construed as weak or strong paternalism. The difference lies in a careful evaluation of patient autonomy, so a PAS request cannot simply be ignored.

Perhaps this is why requests to die are sometimes seen as a manifestation of a common physiological or psychological condition, the symptoms of which are diagnosable and treatable. If the terminal cancer patient and the depressed teenager are similarly psychologically constrained, then in each case the intervention would be an instance of weak, not strong, paternalism. Notice that Rehnquist used the phrase "suicidal impulses." This is a clear indication that PAS requests stem from an underlying cognitive disorder. Aside from any common psychological constraints, the terminal cancer patient must also deal with the raw physical pain of the disease itself. If we regard psychological and physiological pain as common human experiences, then the allegation of false equivalence falls flat: The patient requesting PAS would be easily categorized alongside the teenager contemplating suicide. They are experiencing the same pain both specifically and in general.

Defining pain and suffering in physiological or psychological terms means that it can be managed through pharmaceuticals or therapy. There is some intuitive support for regarding pain in this way. We are accustomed to seeking out motives and intentions for human behavior, so we might try to identify an underlying cause of a patient's desire to die. This desire would be but a symptom or a manifestation of this underlying cause. But there are many problems with this approach to pain and suffering. Construing any desire to die as evidence of a powerful constraint means, by definition, that any intervention will be weakly, not strongly, paternalistic. Is the pain and grief one might experience when confronting one's *own* mortality enough to override autonomy, or is it a rational response to an absurd existential dilemma?

We ignore basic facts of human psychology if we regard all constraints as heteronomous forces. After all, there must be *some* psychological motives for making one decision rather than another. If we care to investigate the patient's actual intentions, we might learn that she is concerned about a loss of self that cannot be accounted for scientifically. This would involve treating her as a person instead of presupposing that all of her values can be reduced to the physiological states of an organism.

Aside from ruling out the possibility of strong paternalism, this medicalization of suffering suggests that we can adequately diagnose and manage its symptoms. But what makes a terminal cancer patient different in kind from a regular patient in therapy is that her suffering can take on an added existential dimension that resists diagnosis and management. Her fear is *objectless* and inexplicable in strictly scientific terms since she is faced with the inevitability of her own nonexistence. For this reason, it seems like a mistake to suggest that her anxiety can be reduced to as a symptom of a deeper physiological or psychological condition.

Being depressed about events that take place in the course of an ordinary life (e.g., health problems, the death of a loved one) seems different in kind from being depressed about not existing at all. Death might not itself be an experience in life, but this does not make it meaningless. It just makes it unintelligible given our ordinary ways of dealing with pain and suffering.

One might argue that the medicalization of suffering is the only available strategy for dealing with end-of-life issues. After all, doctors and nurses cannot have access to the existential suffering of terminal patients. Therefore, they must treat pain in the only way that is available to them: physiologically and psychologically. This response has the virtue of recognizing the dilemma rather than dismissing it. It claims that it would be inappropriate or even impossible to expect doctors and nurses to do more than they are trained to do.

Notice that this is a rather large concession if mortality is a source of nontrivial and even absolute individuation. It grants that end-of-life dilemmas *must* fit within a scientific framework for understanding pain and suffering, even if they are in principle outside the scope of medicine. Daniel Callahan has advanced this argument in various forms. In a fascinating exchange with John Lachs, Callahan stresses the privacy and even the inscrutability of existential suffering at the end of life. But then he concludes that doctors and nurses, having no access to this subjective interpretation of pain, cannot participate in any actions that would cause the death of the patient. In his essay "When Self-Determination Runs Amok," Callahan writes,

> The degree and intensity to which people suffer from their diseases and their dying, and whether they find life more of a burden than a benefit, has very little directly to do with the nature or extent of their actual physical condition. Three people can have the same condition, but only one will find the suffering unbearable. People suffer, but suffering is as much of a function of the values of individuals as it is of the physical causes of that suffering.[17]

In the same article, he describes this desire to die as a "private, idiosyncratic view of the good life" that involves the wish to alienate what must be treated as inalienable: the right to life.[18]

Although this response is provocative, it seems misguided. First, characterizing the values of a terminal patient as idiosyncratic preferences fails to grasp the gravity of this issue. This is especially true if the loss of self caused by disease, aggressive treatment, and sedation is a legitimate concern. Second, if intentions are private and inscrutable, then the legal and moral foundation of the distinction between refusing treatment and requesting to die also collapses. As we see in chapter 3, the legal and moral consensus on these issues depends upon determining the motives of doctors and patients. Palliative sedation is regarded as categorically distinct from physician-assisted suicide because the doctor intends to relieve pain, not kill the patient. If our intentions are in principle unknowable, then this distinction becomes senseless.

Third, any discussion of the subjective nature of suffering would do well to distinguish in principle between the wishes of a possibly autonomous adult and someone who clearly lacks autonomy. For instance, one forceful criticism of the Groningen protocol, which outlines the conditions for legalized infanticide in the Netherlands, relies upon the observation that newborn babies can neither form nor express their wishes.[19] This protocol permits infanticide in cases where the infant is experiencing "unbearable suffering," even if the infant is neither terminally ill nor bound to be in the intensive care unit for life. Under these conditions, it seems like a basic violation of the child's future autonomy to euthanize them, especially when we cannot possibly know how much suffering they might be able to bear.

A terminally ill but consenting adult is clearly in a different position from the Dutch infant. The problem with the Groningen protocol is not the absolute privacy of other minds but the fact that the infant could neither form nor express values in the present moment. Nor do we know how much suffering might be bearable in the future. It is totally unconvincing to claim that the suffering of a competent adult is equally mysterious.

Fourth, establishing a patient's right to life only to make it impossible to alienate such a right is punitive and strange. Patients alienate their right to life every day by refusing treatment, either to let a disease run its course or because a certain treatment violates their conscience. An otherwise-healthy Jehovah's Witness may refuse a blood transfusion against the wishes of the medical establishment. If the right to life were absolutely inalienable, then we would forcibly treat such conscientious objectors. Instead, we recognize that such a right can be alienated (if that is even the proper terminology) under certain conditions.

John Lachs responds to Callahan's arguments in his essay "When Abstract Moralizing Runs Amok." The title, an obvious parody of Callahan's, signals Lachs's wish to consider the context in which end-of-life values are formed. For some patients, the "predicament is not intellectual but existential."[20] Until debates over end-of-life dilemmas move beyond abstract maxims, they will fail to reach patients where their actual interests lie. But the problem with this response is that Callahan readily concedes that suffering at the end of life is existential. He concludes that it is therefore outside the scope of what doctors and nurses may be expected to consider. In this way, the subjective nature of suffering can be used as a reason to disregard the first-person perspective.

Leon Kass echoes Callahan's conclusion when he writes, "Against our confidence in mastery and control, we need to remember that old age and dying are not problems to be solved but human experiences that must be faced."[21] Kass counsels acceptance rather than mastery, but such an ethos runs counter to the immense scientific advances we have made over the past century; the challenge is in drawing a moral line in shifting sands. Also, it is not obvious that more control over the timing of one's death is inconsistent with an attitude of acceptance. If accepting one's fate is not synonymous with *enduring* it, then it seems like the terminal cancer patient requesting a fatal dose of barbiturates is the paragon of acceptance. Perhaps she has transgressed some unseen moral limit by making this request, but every single attempt to save her life up to that point was also undoubtedly an attempt to exercise control.

If we wait long enough, then the patient will have already experienced a loss of self and the ability to request some control over the timing of her death. Continuous sedation until death resolves the existential dilemma: It slowly erodes the self until the burden of nontrivial, absolute individuation dissolves. In the case of an advance directive, we let the document contain the autonomous wishes of the patient who has been sedated past the point of expressing her present wishes. In the case of proxy consent, we permit another person to act as a surrogate. But in either case, we no longer have a patient with the ability to consent.

***

As I have already argued, continuous sedation until death should be seen as the intentional eradication of consciousness that predates the death of the organism. But, from the patient's perspective, the idea of one's organism being "unconsciously alive" might seem absurd. And if CSD is supposed to be a sufficient stand-in for physician-assisted suicide, then what are we to make of the six-month gap between death from PAS and death from CSD *when it comes to the patient's values*? Suppose a patient is diagnosed with stage 4 esophageal cancer. He has consented to several rounds of chemotherapy and radiation, but the cancer has spread to the lymph nodes. His doctor informs him that he has six months to live. If PAS is available to him, then he can begin the rigorous process of obtaining a fatal dose of barbiturates. If, however, he is told that he does not need PAS because CSD will eventually end his unbearable pain, then he still has six more months on the downward slope.

In this specific case, the medical, legal, and ethical consensus governing end-of-life scenarios seems seriously inadequate. As I noted, the Uniform Determination of Death Act (UDDA) is a standard that we can generally use to ensure consistency in patient care at the end of life. Defining death as the complete cessation of brain activity or cardiopulmonary function is usually a reasonable standard. However, the fact that this consensus has emerged does not mean that it should apply in all cases. Uniformity does not entail objectivity, even if we often fail to recognize this.

In their book *Defining Death: The Case for Choice*, Robert Veatch and Lainie Ross give credence to the higher-brain definition of death, which states that an irreversible loss of consciousness is a sufficient condition for death.[22] They argue that patients should have some degree of choice between competing definitions (whole-brain death, cardiopulmonary death, and higher-brain death) based on their own personal values. One might not wish to muddle up what we normally think is an easily diagnosed condition (i.e., death). But there is no avoiding the fact that scientific and ethical expertise cannot definitively resolve this question. And if it is unpalatable to offer patients the choice between competing definitions of death, then they could still make an informed choice about whether consciousness and the organism perish simultaneously or in phases. So we need not resolve the question of when one *really* dies in order to recognize the dilemma generated from having continuous sedation as an inevitable outcome.

The obvious problem here is that empirical advances generate new problems that are not themselves strictly empirical. For instance, we can medically induce a coma and cool the body considerably to reduce brain swelling. But nothing about our scientific ability to do this can tell us whether it should be done *in any particular case.* No system of scientific claims can definitively resolve this question for the patient. And in the case of some end-of-life dilemmas, no amount of ethical debate among those with putative expertise can settle the issue.

In the context of end-of-life issues, we often fall victim to a "false sense of scientific objectivity."[23] Mark Wicclair coins this phrase to criticize our deferential attitude in debates over futility. It is immediately assumed that doctors must be experts in determining whether a procedure is futile. However, futility can take on multiple meanings, depending on what perspective one adopts. For example, a 2 percent chance that CPR will revive my loved one is physiologically futile, but it might not be futile from the standpoint of a patient's goals. In this case, 2 percent is *infinitely* better than 0 percent. A doctor might still decide to stop resuscitating the patient, but that involves a difficult judgment call. It is a simple act of self-deception to believe that the doctor's judgment could be sanctioned by invoking a magic word. And since the judgment about whether a treatment is futile admits of no certainty, we should be equally careful about deferring to ethical expertise.

When it comes to defining and diagnosing death, we tend to act as if this were simply an empirical question. Recall that our current standard involves either the death of the whole brain or a complete cessation of cardiopulmonary function. The notion that an irreversible loss of consciousness could signal the death of the patient seems too speculative and unverifiable. The underlying assumption here is that a physiological definition is required because death is no doubt a biological phenomenon. Our determination of death should be scientifically demonstrable instead of depending upon the judgment of a doctor.

However, if we take this line of argument to its logical conclusion, then the best standard of death that we could hope for would be total organ failure or even complete cell death. This definition is unambiguous and perfectly physiological. No one, however, accepts this definition in practice. If we did, then we would no longer be able to harvest healthy organs for transplantation. In a society incapable of, or unconcerned with, organ donation, total organ failure (or even complete cell death) would constitute a better biological definition. This suggests that the extent to which we employ a physiological determination of death is largely a function of our societal values and technological capabilities.

The whole-brain standard attempts to strike a compromise between our values and our need for a properly biological definition. The patient is dead if and only if the entire brain (including the brain stem) has ceased to function. This means that organs can still be harvested, so our values are preserved. It also means that the *organism* is dead, so the definition is still biologically based. The death of the organism, on this view, predates the death of the entire body, insofar as one's organs can still be healthy and functioning.

So what seemed to be a clear definition has become more complicated: The death of organism is not synonymous with complete physiological death. Rather, proponents of this definition have *judged* that the brain is the key unifying factor in making raw biological material into an organism. If this is so, then an inquiry that purported to be merely empirical must now have its ontological claim defended. We need some reason to believe that a patient is dead once the entire brain is dead and not before (which would be too speculative) or after (which would conflict with our values).

For this reason, it is disingenuous to claim that the whole-brain view is properly empirical, while competing definitions of death (e.g., the irreversible loss of consciousness) are not. The question of when a patient is dead is inextricably tied up with our technological abilities, our societal values, and our reasoned judgment. If this is so, then conflating the following two propositions is a serious category mistake: 1) It is a scientific fact that the patient is dead, and 2) judged by the whole-brain definition of death, the patient is dead. The first proposition is senseless on its own since there is no purely scientific definition. Or if there is, it would have to include total organ failure or complete cell death. When the first claim is provided context in the second statement, we can now judge whether it is true. For instance, we could test for activity in the brain stem. But we still require a reason for adopting that standard in the first place, and that is something that science cannot provide.

This is the same problem as determining whether a procedure is futile. Unfortunately, there is no neutral standpoint on this question. Judged physiologically, the procedure is futile. Judged from the perspective of patient goals, it might not be.

In addition to requiring a judgment about what makes biological material into an organism, our diagnosis of death is intimately connected to the question of the moral status of the patient. For instance, we diagnose death to know whether we can pull the plug on someone on life support. We devise a "dead donor rule" for organ harvesting so that a transplant does not *kill* the donor.[24] Here, too, the whole-brain approach must walk a fine line: If we diagnose death too early, then the act of harvesting organs has killed the patient. But if we wait too long, we run the risk of healthy organs deteriorating before they can find a new home. There is some irony in the fact that a person can be declared dead from cardiac arrest and have that same heart function in another human being.[25] On the other hand, a patient awaiting a heart transplant might not get a healthy one if the whole-brain diagnosis is made too late. So we cannot avoid questions of judgment and moral status in the determination of death.

James Bernat, a well-known proponent of the whole-brain definition of death, acknowledges some of these conceptual problems.[26] He also admits that whole-brain death may, in fact, be improperly diagnosed. This concession echoes a persistent problem with the way in which this standard is used in hospitals. Although it purports to be a uniform determination of death, there is very little uniformity in how it is determined and enforced. In spite of this practical problem, however, Bernat maintains that the whole-brain standard is the best definition for public policy purposes. He worries that adopting the higher-brain standard would undermine the confidence of the public. It would permit far too many false positives, and it would counterintuitively regard death as a speculative conceptual question rather than a biological fact.

On Bernat's view, the whole-brain definition is empirically superior to other views, even if it requires the judgment that the brain is physiologically essential. He develops this argument with reference to an idea proposed by Jacques Loeb in 1916: "Loeb explained that organisms are not simply composites of cells, tissues, and organs, but possess overarching functions that regulate and integrate all systems to maintain the unity and interrelatedness of the organism."[27] For something to count as an organism, it must have *organization* as an emergent function. As Bernat explains, "An emergent function is a property of a whole that is not possessed by any of its component parts, and that cannot be reduced to one or more of its component parts."[28] Over time, cells gain specialized functions, individual organs form an integrated system, and an organism emerges as something ontologically unique. For this reason, we can define death as the irreversible loss of what makes an organism *what it is*.

There are a few problems with these claims, however. One minor complaint is that any individual organ we harvest from someone diagnosed as brain dead is itself a functioning system of cells. We can even harvest a heart, liver, and a kidney simultaneously, all of which exhibit emergent functions. As for the organism itself, Bernat is claiming that the entire brain, including the brain stem, has to be dead in order for a *generalized* emergent function to be obsolete. But what if consciousness is central to the type of emergent function that Bernat deems necessary for an organism to exist *as* an organism? As Oliver Burkeman writes,

> A team of researchers led by [Giulio] Tononi has designed a device that stimulates the brain with electrical voltage, to measure how interconnected and organised—how "integrated"—its neural circuits are. Sure enough, when people fall into a deep sleep, or receive an injection of anaesthetic, as they slip into unconsciousness, the device demonstrates that their brain integration declines, too. Among patients suffering "locked-in syndrome"—who are as conscious as the rest of us—levels of brain integration remain high; among patients in coma—who aren't—it doesn't.[29]

If these findings are plausible, then the whole-brain view might ultimately collapse into the higher-brain model (i.e., irreversible loss of consciousness). In other words, if the brain is what produces the organism (via emergent function), then perhaps a key feature of the brain (consciousness) is what permits it to do this. Or, at the very least, consciousness would increase the degree to which an organism exhibits the type of emergent function that we claim to value.

In this way, those who defend the whole-brain standard might ultimately be committed to declaring an organism dead, even though areas like the brain stem still function. At the very least, this research suggests that claims about consciousness are not vague and speculative. They are biologically based, just as the whole-brain view prides itself on being empirical. Robert Veatch defends the higher-brain model in this way, arguing that the integration of bodily and mental function is critical to a human being alive.[30] Note that this argument has *nothing* to do with claims about a patient's quality of life; it simply recognizes the contribution of consciousness to the overall integration of an organism.

Both the whole-brain and the higher-brain models involve judgments about what is necessary for an organism to emerge and to die. As neuroscience and medical technology advance, so, too, will our ability to diagnose the irreversible loss of consciousness. We might also be able to determine more precisely how consciousness contributes to the integrated functioning of an organism. In this way, some objections about incorporating consciousness into a definition of death may be met simply with better technology.

But regardless of any future scientific advancements in understanding consciousness, it is already clear that we do not take a patient's conscious confrontation with mortality seriously enough. We fail to recognize this problem of informed consent because we intuitively defer to the current conceptual framework governing end-of-life dilemmas. By this logic, a patient who is administered continuous sedation until death is not even a *candidate* for informed consent. Instead, we should recognize that our policies and procedures created the conditions for the patient being passively sedated into permanent unconsciousness.

***

Our willingness to defer to scientific and ethical expertise signals our unwillingness, or even our inability, to think about a *particular* individual. Any concern for patient values is usually framed in terms of the rules, policies, and procedures stipulated by a legal and moral consensus. But framing the issue in this way is the opposite mistake of viewing patient values as private and idiosyncratic preferences. For instance, if Ms. Bouvia had clarified that her desire to refuse treatment was not a generalizable opinion about all patients with cerebral palsy, the court would have ignored her. It was required to identify the right rule to apply, and this necessarily deals with generalities rather than specifics. Once a patient is sorted into the appropriate group, there is no legal or moral permission to opt out of it. This is true even if one's own mortality is at issue.

Legal and moral verdicts are general in their very nature, requiring the affirmation of some essential similarity between distinct cases. Adopting this legal or moral attitude toward individual cases is, under normal conditions, not a problem. Comparing and contrasting particular cases and debating whether general rules ever admit of individual exceptions is a common and intelligible activity. However, might end-of-life decisions be a strange and singular exception to this way of thinking?

Why is the move from the particular (where end-of-life values are formed) to the general or even universal (where legal and moral verdicts are rendered) and back to the particular (where permission to die is granted or denied) sensible in the first place? Here is the heart of the dilemma: Can this nontrivial form of individuation be understood within a legal and moral framework, in spite of the fact that it requires the adoption of a completely different and even incommensurable point of view? If so, then how is this possible? If not, then does this reveal a basic but profound limitation in how we frame end-of-life decisions?

In a sense, these questions invert the traditional Kantian project of discovering the conditions for a universal morality. Kant's basic metaethical project explored the conditions for the possibility of making absolute moral judgments of one another.[31] For him, the moral *ought* was issued as a categorical imperative, a universal command. But what is so interesting about end-of-life decisions, if they arise from a nontrivial and even absolute form of individuation, is that they pose the opposite problem. How does one get from the first-person perspective to the third-person point of view (a legal and moral framework) without simply begging the question about the authority of legal and moral judgments? If these judgments are authoritative, can they also be adequately justified? And what form should this justification take?

The dangers of generalizing and thinking abstractly about a specific ethical dilemma are ever present. It is natural to want to draw general conclusions from particular observations, but doing this in the context of end-of-life dilemmas is misleading. Our rules, policies, and procedures compel us to classify and categorize, to recognize (or invent) commonalities. Even the language we use in doing so is general rather than particular. In order to form and communicate concepts at all, we must first distill out individual differences so that we can generalize. Elizabeth Bouvia is transformed into the *Bouvia* case. We talk about *patients* with common symptoms and prognoses, so this kind of abstract thinking seeps down into our grammar.

Sometimes a suggestive play on words effectively makes this point: The Cleveland Clinic promoted a centennial campaign called "The Power of Every *One*."[32] It is a clever slogan: *Everyone* is the universal concept, and every *one* obviously refers to each particular individual. The challenge, though, is in finding a way to actually think about particular patients, constrained as we are by our principles (and our language in general) to classify and categorize.

When Oliver Sacks, the physician and professor of neurology, learned that had terminal cancer, he wrote a short essay titled "My Own Life."[33] This is the same title as David Hume's autobiography, written on a single day in April 1776.[34] In this short book, Hume recounts his attitude toward his own mortality after learning he was gravely ill. Dr. Sacks shares some of Hume's sentiments, but he also points out some key differences in their dispositions. His ironic use of Hume's title captures the sense in which mortality is a common experience but also ultimately and absolutely one's own. The problem is that we do not seem very well equipped legally, morally, and even conceptually and linguistically to think about particular individuals confronting their own mortality.

Moral harm can be imposed on individuals when we fail to recognize our tendency to think abstractly. A severe but instructive example of this can be found in a quote attributed to Josef Stalin: "One death is a tragedy; one million is a statistic."[35] Abel Herzberg, a Holocaust survivor, passionately inverted the dictator's logic when he claimed, "There were not six million Jews murdered; there was one murder, six million times."[36]

Their disagreement is ontological, not just moral, since they are counting individuals differently. Herzberg is undoubtedly right on the merits, but he might be asking us to do the impossible. If the very concepts we rely on to think and communicate trade in universals rather than particulars, then it will be hard to imagine, much less mourn, six million murdered individuals. End-of-life dilemmas compound this problem for two reasons: First, they are rife with legal and moral ambiguity instead of being morally unambiguous like the Holocaust. Second, they involve the first-person perspective of the person facing self-extinction; the patient is not a victim of violence.

Medical ethicists have, for the most part, avoided asking these types of questions about this paradigmatic existential issue. Formulating rules, policies, and procedures to govern end-of-life dilemmas presupposes the authority of scientific and ethical insight. But the careful legal and moral distinctions we have carved out to resolve these dilemmas underwrite a suspicious ontology of the patient. These distinctions cannot relieve us of the increasing burden of choice, and they cannot save us from our mortal condition. Our principles cannot answer the question of whether it is better to exercise some control over the manner and timing of one's death or to perish in a narcotic stupor. If answers to these kinds of questions are outside the scope of medicine, the law, and even modern medical ethics, then I suppose that is the point.

NOTES

1. Leo Tolstoy, *The Death of Ivan Ilyich*, trans. Lynn Solotaroff (New York: Bantam Dell, 1981), 113.
2. Fyodor Dostoevsky, *The Idiot*, trans. David McDuff (Penguin: Amazon Digital Services, 2004), 72.
3. Dostoevsky, *The Idiot*, 72.
4. Dostoevsky's *The House of the Dead* is a semi-autobiographical account of his time in a Siberian prison camp (New York: Dover, 2004).
5. For a unique perspective on the afterlife, see Samuel Scheffler: *Death and the Afterlife* (New York: Oxford University Press, 2013).
6. National Geographic Channel, "Funeral Strippers," *Taboo Video*, accessed August 3, 2016, http://channel.nationalgeographic.com/taboo/videos/funeral-strippers/.
7. For some provocative analysis of this moral dilemma, see Peter Unger, *Living High and Letting Die: Our Illusion of Innocence* (New York: Oxford University Press, 1996). In his own damning editorial, Peter Singer approvingly cites Unger. See "The Singer Solution to World Poverty," *New York Times*, September 5, 1999.
8. For some reflections on how to treat this illness, see John Portman, "Pneumonia, Friend of the Elderly," *Western Journal of Medicine* 173, no. 4 (October 2000): 277-78.
9. Mike Scott, "For Steve Gleason and Family, New Documentary Is 'As Real as It Can Get,'" July 22, 2016, accessed July 23, 2016, http://www.nola.com/movies/index.ssf/2016/07/steve_gleason_documentary_mich.html.
10. *Bouvia v. Superior Court* 225 Cal Rpt. 297 (Cal. App 2d Dist 1986).
11. Vicki Michel points out the question-begging nature of arguments in defense of non-terminal patients refusing treatment. See her "Suicide by Persons with Disabilities Disguised as the Refusal of Life-Sustaining Treatment," *HEC Forum* 7 (1995): 122-31.
12. Chief Justice William H. Rehnquist, opinion of the court in *Washington v. Glucksberg*, U.S. Supreme Court, 521 U.S. 702 (1997).
13. For an interesting legal analysis of this concept, see Kenneth I. Winston, "On Treating Like Cases Alike," *California Law Review*. 62/1 (1974).

14. See Leanne J. Fisher, "The Suicide Trap: *Bouvia v. Superior Court* and the Right to Refuse Medical Treatment," *Loyola of Los Angeles Law Review*. 219/21 (1987).

15. The most famous of these critics is Immanuel Kant, who argues that suicide is inherently irrational. See Kant's *Lectures on Ethics*, ed. and trans. Peter Heath (Cambridge: Cambridge University Press, 1997), 144-49.

16. See Terrence F. Ackerman, "Why Doctors Should Intervene," *Hastings Center Report* 12 (1982): 14-17.

17. Daniel Callahan, "When Self-Determination Runs Amok," *Hastings Center Report* 22, no. 2 (1992): 53.

18. Callahan, "When Self-Determination Runs Amok," 52.

19. See Edward Verhagen and Pieter J. J. Sauer, "The Groningen Protocol—Euthanasia in Severely Ill Newborns," *New England Journal of Medicine* 352, no. 10 (2005): 959-62.

20. John Lachs, "When Abstract Moralizing Runs Amok," *Journal of Clinical Ethics* 5, no. 1 (1994): 10-13.

21. Leon Kass, "Lingering Longer: Who Will Care?" *Washington Post*, September 29, 2005, accessed May 23, 2016, http://www.washingtonpost.com/wpdyn/content/article/2005/09/28/AR2005092802119.html.

22. Robert Veatch and Lainie Ross, *Defining Death: The Case for Choice* (Washington D.C.: Georgetown University Press, 2016).

23. Mark Wicclair, *Ethics and the Elderly* (Oxford: Oxford University Press, 1993), 28.

24. For a compelling discussion of this protocol, see Robert Truog and Franklin Miller, "The Dead Donor Rule and Organ Transplantation," *New England Journal of Medicine* 359 (2008): 674-75.

25. See Robert Veatch, "Donating Hearts after Cardiac Death—Reversing the Irreversible," *New England Journal of Medicine* 359 (2008): 672-73.

26. James Bernat, "The Whole-Brain Concept of Death Remains Optimum Public Policy," *Journal of Law, Medicine, and Ethics* 34, no. 1 (2006): 35-43.

27. Bernat, "Whole-Brain Concept," 38.

28. Bernat, "Whole-Brain Concept," 38.

29. Oliver Burkeman, "Why Can't the World's Greatest Minds Solve the Mystery of Consciousness?" January 21, 2015, accessed November 1, 2015, https://www.theguardian.com/science/2015/jan/21/-sp-why-cant-worlds-greatest-minds-solve-mystery-consciousness.

30. See especially Robert Veatch, "The Death of Whole-Brain Death: The Plague of the Disaggregators, Somaticists, and Mentalists," *Journal of Medicine and Philosophy* 30, no. 4 (2005): 353-78.

31. This is especially true in Immanuel Kant, *Groundwork for the Metaphysics of Morals*, trans. Mary Gregor and Jens Timmermann (Cambridge: Cambridge University Press, 2012).

32. Cleveland Clinic, "The Power of Every One," *Centennial Campaign*, accessed June 16, 2015, http://giving.clevelandclinic.org/articles/power-every-one.

33. Oliver Sacks, "My Own Life," *New York Times*, February 19, 2015, accessed October 2, 2015, http://www.nytimes.com/2015/02/19/opinion/oliver-sacks-on-learning-he-has-terminal-cancer.html?_r=0.

34. David Hume, "My Own Life," April 18, 1776, accessed July 29, 2015, http://isites.harvard.edu/fs/docs/icb.topic880131.files/My.Own.Life.by.David.Hume.pdf.

35. This quote is apocryphal, and its source is unclear and contested. On my view, it does not matter who originally articulated this profound concept. The sentiment remains the same.

36. See Abel Herzberg, "The Holocaust: Crimes, Heroes, and Villains," accessed January 4, 2015, http://www.auschwitz.dk/.

Part II

Chapter Three

Using and Abusing the Doctrine of Double Effect

On June 5, 1944, General Dwight D. Eisenhower must have been the loneliest person in the world. As supreme commander of Operation Overlord, he was responsible for launching the largest amphibious attack in history. The decision to invade Normandy was gut-wrenching for a variety of reasons. Aside from the fact that it promised to be extraordinarily bloody even if it were successful, factors outside of the general's control could doom the mission completely.

Two variables worth mentioning are 1) the painstaking effort to deceive the Nazis into believing that the invasion would occur elsewhere and 2) something as simple as the weather. If the Nazis knew where the invasion was to take place, they would massacre the Allied troops. But even if they were caught off guard, a bad break in the weather would prove to be catastrophic. Only a few days in June promised the perfect combination of cloud cover and clear views. If the weather were too clear, then the Nazis would be able to spot the invasion from miles away. On the other hand, if visibility were too diminished, then there would be insufficient air support for the troops on the beaches.

On the night before the invasion, the general toured the camps. He shook hands with the men whose fate he, in large part, determined. Hopeful, but with a heavy heart, Eisenhower made the final call to invade. He could foresee with certainty that thousands of his men would die. Still, he accepted full responsibility for making the decision.[1]

On June 26, 1997, the Supreme Court issued a verdict in the case *Vacco v. Quill*. They upheld New York's ban on physician-assisted suicide, writing the following: "The law has long used actors' intent or purpose to distinguish between two acts that may have the same result. Put differently, the law distinguishes actions taken ‘because of’ a given end from actions taken ‘in spite of’ their unintended but foreseen consequences.”[2]

Then the court provided an example, quoting an excerpt from the lower court’s verdict in this case: “When General Eisenhower ordered American soldiers onto the beaches of Normandy, he knew that he was sending many American soldiers to certain death. . . . His purpose, though, was to . . . liberate Europe from the Nazis.”[3]

The difference between foreseen and *intended* consequences as opposed to foreseen but *unintended* consequences is legally and morally critical. It has come to be known as the doctrine of double effect (hereafter DDE). This principle explains why General Eisenhower is not morally responsible for the deaths of Allied soldiers, even though he commanded them to invade Normandy. Based on the court’s logic, it also explains the absolute difference between physician-assisted suicide and continuous sedation until death. One death is both foreseen and intended, while the other is foreseen but not intended.

In the last chapter, I discussed the many reasons we have demonstrated an unwillingness, or even an inability, to think about a *particular* individual confronting end-of-life dilemmas. I focused on the significance of a patient’s conscious experience of this dilemma and how our current conceptual framework obscures this. I challenged our tacit (or even explicit) endorsement of scientific and ethical expertise, and I suggested that our obsession with policy formulation seeps into the very language we use to discuss end-of-life dilemmas.

In this chapter, I evaluate the DDE, the key legal and moral principle that undergirds the distinction between physician-assisted suicide and continuous sedation until death. My concern here is that there are too many epistemological problems with applying this general principle to end-of-life dilemmas. This includes questions concerning patient and doctor intent, the challenge of isolating a specific cause of death, and our inability to claim that inducing a permanent loss of consciousness is proportionate to eradicating pain. I conclude by arguing that the “devil’s choice” is a more honest explanatory model for end-of-life choices when compared with the doctrine of double effect.

As a general ethical principle, the DDE helps us determine whether someone should be held responsible for an action that may produce an undesirable outcome or even serious harm. Here is the most basic version of the principle: It can be legally and morally permissible for one’s action to cause harm but only if the action directly produces a good result, while the harm produced is a foreseen but unintended side effect. Further, the harm produced must be proportionate to (and not exceed) the good outcome. Some versions of the DDE also include the requirement that the action be designed to restore a status quo that has been upended. For instance, one can use reasonable force to defend oneself from harm, but this does not include an excessive and vindictive use of force. Nor does it mean that one is entitled to use force indefinitely.

This concept has been used to explain the difference between suicide and heroic sacrifice, between the deliberate targeting of civilians and the accidental death of an innocent bystander, and between physician-assisted suicide and continuous sedation until death. The doctrine of double effect is one of the main ethical principles in support of continuous sedation until death, and it is the chief source of legal and moral condemnation of physician-assisted suicide. CSD is legitimate because it foresees but does not intend the death of the patient, whereas PAS is illicit because it both foresees and intends the patient's death.

I readily admit that this principle captures something intuitive about the nature of legal and moral responsibility. As such, it can be successfully defended against a utilitarian criticism that suggests that we care only about outcomes and not intent. Two events might produce similarly bad outcomes, but it does not follow that they generate the same degree of blame. For instance, there is a clear difference between deliberately targeting and accidentally killing a civilian. While the phrase "collateral damage" sounds insensitive, the fact that the death was not intentionally caused is legally and morally significant.

In spite of its usefulness, the DDE raises some significant questions about appealing to agent intent and causation. These two concepts are notoriously complicated, so it is a little strange that, together, they form the basis of a dominant legal and moral principle. Let us begin with the question of determining intent. This term immediately takes on two different meanings: whether the action was done deliberately and whether one willed the outcome of the action. In the context of the DDE, it is necessary but not sufficient for an agent to have deliberately made the decision. One must also have willed the outcome.

Here is a real-life example from several years ago.[4] A husband is driving down the highway with his pregnant wife in the passenger seat. He sees an SUV traveling in the wrong direction, and he knows that it will strike their car in a matter of moments. The husband decides to turn the wheel so that he will take the full force of the collision, hoping that his pregnant wife might be spared. His plans works, his wife survives, and the baby was born healthy. No one would call this a case of suicide, even though the husband deliberately turned the wheel. That is because he was not motivated to die, even though he could foresee this outcome with near certainty. So this is a case of heroic sacrifice, not suicide.

The distinction between an action done deliberately and an action whose outcome is also endorsed is clear in this case. But in spite of the fact that the DDE stipulates that foreseeing and intending are categorically distinct elements of the same action, there are many cases where this is not so clear. Take, for instance, any action where an agent deliberately chooses to do something that she knows to be harmful to herself. If the DDE is correct, then she can plausibly claim not to intend the self-inflicted harm, even though she can foresee to a high degree that it will come to pass. Cigarette smokers are not slowly committing suicide because they only intend a delicious nicotine high. Despite repeated warnings from a doctor, one cannot commit suicide by binging on fat and sugar, so long as one only intends short-term pleasure.

In these cases, we have good reason to wonder whether foreseeing and intending are categorically distinct or whether foreseeing can bleed into intending. Sometimes a high degree of foreknowledge seems reasonably correlated with an intention to bring about that result. Or at the very least, it seems correlated with a willingness to discount the future. Suppose that a cigarette smoker with lung cancer in her family history were warned to stop smoking. She responds to the dire warning by indicating her disinterest in dying at the age of ninety in a nursing home. In this case, she is willing to sacrifice years that she presumes she would not enjoy living.

Whether we wish to call this suicide or not, this admission is a strong indication that her motive matches her deliberate decision. She is willing to sacrifice her future self for the sake of present enjoyment. Notice how the example changes if the smoker confesses that she is hopelessly addicted to nicotine. We would *not* attribute the same motivation in this case.

Sometimes we attribute a "death wish" to an individual who undertakes especially risky behavior. But even *this* does not really rise to the level of suicidal ideation. Intent, in such a case, serves as a moral shield against accusations of ultimate recklessness. Sometimes an adoring public even praises wanton self-disregard as heroism, even as they anticipate (and hope?) that the worst might in fact happen.[5] This suggests that intent, for the DDE, is sacrosanct, while merely foreseeing entails no real moral consequences.

If this is true, then an intuitively plausible principle can easily be perverted into something quite different. Someone can willfully and repeatedly risk his life but be accused of nothing stronger than having a death wish. On the other hand, a terminal cancer patient who desperately wants to live but chooses PAS over CSD is committing suicide. One person has deliberately put herself in a position where she might lose her life, whereas the other is horrified to find herself in that position. Now suppose that the risky behavior is being exhibited by someone who is still quite young. According to the DDE, the willful discounting of her (considerable) future carries no serious moral weight, whereas the terminal cancer patient is wrong to risk losing six months of foreseeable suffering.

Other examples call into question the very possibility of suicidal intent. They do not show how foreseeing to such a high degree might be correlated with an intention. Rather, they challenge the possibility that an agent could meaningfully intend the action that she has deliberately chosen. Two examples come to mind: CTE (chronic traumatic encephalopathy) and PTSD (post-traumatic stress disorder). A disturbing number of professional athletes who have experienced severe brain damage have killed themselves. Likewise, a shocking percentage of combat veterans kill themselves upon returning home. Both conditions challenge the way in which we conceptualize suicide.

Dave Duerson's story is a case in point. He was a Super Bowl-winning enforcer on perhaps the best defense ever: The 1985 Chicago Bears. Later in life he continued his success as a respected businessman and a beloved husband and father. However, his temperament abruptly changed, and his life completely fell apart. Dave shot himself through the chest, requesting in a note that his brain be donated for scientific study. He was posthumously diagnosed with CTE, a neurodegenerative disorder that explains his sudden and dramatic decline. So far, 96 percent of NFL players whose brains have been examined have been diagnosed with this affliction.[6] Our scientific understanding of PTSD is, I would argue, less advanced at this point. What is clear, though, is that the war does not end even when the mission is completed. The number of combat veterans who return home and take their own lives is nauseatingly high.[7]

According to the DDE, someone has committed suicide if and only if they both foresaw and intended that outcome. As we have already seen, intent cannot simply refer to something done deliberately. Otherwise, the husband who saved his pregnant wife by turning the wheel committed suicide. So intent must also mean that the agent was sufficiently motivated to end her life. But cases of CTE and PTSD suggest that agent intention might be even more complicated than that. There is some cruel irony in the fact that Mr. Duerson reasonably (and correctly) suspected that his brain was irrevocably damaged. It would be preposterous to suggest that Dave would have willed any of the bad events that destroyed his life. But it would be equally strange to claim that he willed his own demise, were it not for the condition that afflicted him. So if intent cannot only mean something done deliberately, perhaps it is similarly superficial to say that it means something actively willed by the agent.

In cases like these, the concept of intent needs to be either discarded or seriously reformed. One way to salvage it might be to consider the agent's reflective awareness of his or her desires. If we adopt what has been called an "endorsement constraint,"[8] then we would care whether the person could critically endorse and identify with the values expressed in his desires and, ultimately, in his actions. For instance, one might have violent tendencies that perhaps even manifest in violent actions. When it comes to questions of moral praise and blame, however, we might care a lot about the reflective attitude that one holds about the disposition that one happens to have. In this case, we might morally distinguish between someone attempting to control his impulses and someone who hurts people unrepentantly. Likewise, someone could be genetically predisposed to craving alcohol, but perhaps it is the person's reflective attitude about that craving that matters. We would be right to praise a recovering alcoholic for maintaining sobriety, and we would be mistaken for commending a teetotaler who never experienced a craving at all.

If we take the idea of an endorsement constraint seriously, then the DDE becomes more compelling but far more complex. Its usefulness was, in a way, entailed by its simplicity. If it matters to us that Dave explicitly recognized his neurodegenerative condition, then we might *deny* that he would have reflectively endorsed the action of putting a gun to his chest and pulling the trigger. So the evidence that he intended to die would need to be stronger than the fact that he did it deliberately or that he was sufficiently motivated by a desire to pull the trigger at that time. We would have to know if he could reflectively and critically identify with the desire to shoot himself.

If we care about Dave's reflective attitude toward the situation in which he found himself, then claims about suicide require a high evidential burden. In his case, we have a note indicating his wishes and (arguably) implying a sense of remorse that his life came to this point. But in most examples, we do not have sufficient information for judging someone's reflective attitude. This lack of insight means that we should tread lightly when labeling an action as a suicide.

Unfortunately, it is clear that we exercise no such caution in our discussions of physician-assisted suicide. In chapter 2, I discussed an obvious false equivalence between a terminal cancer patient self-administering a fatal dose of barbiturates and a depressed but otherwise healthy teenager who commits suicide. The conditions that give rise to the desire to end one's own life are absolutely different. Any effort to equate the two desires by showing how they manifest the same underlying psychological symptoms is, I think, intellectually dishonest. And yet we pay little attention to the extent to which a terminal cancer patient satisfies the endorsement constraint. Doing so would seriously mitigate our ability to ascribe suicidal intent. It would also challenge the straightforward use of the DDE to render a verdict about licit and illicit death.

Brittany Maynard, the twenty-nine-year-old California woman stricken with terminal cancer, had a deep urge to continue living. Tragically, she was afflicted with a rare and aggressive form of brain cancer. She moved to Oregon in order to qualify for PAS, and she deliberately self-administered the fatal dose. None of this shows, however, that she was suicidal *in the same way* as someone who reflectively approves of his own desire to die. Instead, Ms. Maynard's case is akin to Mr. Duerson's or to the example of a PTSD-afflicted army lieutenant who kills himself upon returning home. Perhaps it is even clearer than Mr. Duerson's: She knew what was coming for her imminently, whereas Mr. Duerson might have lived many years with his affliction. If the DDE cannot account for cases like Ms. Maynard's, then perhaps it has been misapplied in end-of-life dilemmas.

***

Even if one believes that the DDE offers a sensible account of agent intention, it still fails to provide an adequate description of causality. In a case of heroic sacrifice, where the outcome is foreseen but not intended, we deem the context in which the agent finds himself to be morally significant. For instance, the soldier jumps on the grenade not to commit suicide but to save his brothers. The husband happens to find himself in a dire situation where an oncoming semitruck is about to annihilate his family. The cause of their actions cannot be found solely in what they did but rather in the situation to which they were responding.

As I argued in chapter 2, however, critics of PAS abstract away from the context that makes the desire to die meaningful (i.e., terminal illness with less than six months to live). They focus solely on the isolated decisions of the patient (who requests) and the doctor (who assists). So the patient and the doctor are separately and jointly responsible for the death, and that is where the analysis ends. This discrepancy surfaced in the earlier discussion of CTE and PTSD. If suicide is supposed to involve intentional self-annihilation, then it must be caused by the agent herself. But just as there are strong reasons to question the assumption that Mr. Duerson committed suicide in a conventional sense, the same reasons hold for terminal cancer patients. Terminal illness creates the conditions under which a patient deliberately chooses to die but does not reflectively endorse this attitude. This does not at all mitigate patient consent since the patient freely acknowledges what she is doing and chooses to self-administer the dose. Yet, all things being equal, she does not want to die. She is in the same situation as the man driving down the highway: *Now the semitruck headed in the wrong direction is an overwhelming number of mutated cells attacking her body.* The fact that the man and his family would die imminently does not make this example categorically distinct from the terminal cancer patient. Whether it is six seconds or six months, the important point is that both deaths are inevitable.

For these reasons, it is overly reductive to suppose that PAS involves two isolated choices (the patient's request and the doctor's assistance). Having labeled it a suicide, it is understandable that we would make this mistake. This way of framing the issue demands that we find a clear and specific cause of death, even though we acknowledge complexity in cases of heroic sacrifice. Otherwise we would not be able to easily distinguish between a patient being killed and a patient being allowed to die. But the easy answer is not always correct, and we cannot always rely on our definition of suicide to render simple verdicts.

Occasionally we are willing to examine more closely the conditions under which someone causes their own death. We are sometimes even willing to grant causal efficacy to these conditions instead of isolating an individual's deliberate decision as the sole cause. For instance, in the wake of the attacks on 9/11, the New York City medical examiner's office had to determine the cause of death for roughly two hundred people who jumped from the Twin Towers. They classified these deaths as "homicide by blunt force trauma" rather than suicide. A spokesperson for the office defended this judgment: "Jumping indicates a choice, and these people did not have that choice. That is why the deaths were ruled homicide, because the actions of other people caused them to die."[9]

The medical examiners should be commended for their willingness to recognize the causal complexity involved in the decision to jump from a burning building. However, it is fair to ask whether the reluctance to label these deaths as suicides stemmed from a desire to avoid adding moral blame to an already terrible event. It was bad enough that these people died in this way; there was no need to compile the pain by accusing them of committing suicide.

This suggests that our causal determinations are stained and colored by our moral sense. Labeling something as a suicide is just not a straightforward causal claim; it entails a strong moral judgment, too. So the DDE does not offer us a clear and impartial way of determining intention and causation. We make exceptions when we want to avoid making a strong moral judgment or when we want to emphatically judge an action as heroic. But what exactly is the difference between someone jumping from a burning building and a terminal cancer patient self-administering a fatal dose?

The example I used to begin this chapter perfectly illustrates the way in which our moral judgments cloud our causal claims. On the court's view, General Eisenhower foresaw but did not intend the deaths of thousands of Allied soldiers on D-Day. Those deaths were a regrettable but indirect consequence of the decision to invade. It is telling that the Supreme Court would cherry-pick such an emotionally charged example. No one would deny that those deaths were both tragic and heroic. Nor would anyone deny the moral righteousness of Eisenhower's intention to liberate Europe from the Nazis.

But even this clear application of the DDE leaves us with some lingering questions. Suppose that any number of factors turned a successful invasion into a massacre on the beach. I already mentioned the significance of the weather and the counterintelligence campaign. What if Rommel had not decided to take a minivacation to celebrate his wife's birthday?[10] What if Hitler had suddenly decided to break his strange habit of oversleeping and commanding his officers not to wake him? Hundreds of variables produced a successful invasion, and a change in any one of these elements could have led to a completely different outcome. Yet the DDE isolates one moment in time, abstracting it from the context that made it meaningful.

If the mission had been an abject failure, Eisenhower's attitude toward planning it might now seem qualitatively different. Before the invasion, Eisenhower wrote, "The operation is not being planned with any alternatives. This operation is planned as a victory, and that's the way it's going to be. We're going down there, and we're throwing everything we have into it, and we're going to make it a success."[11] If the plan succeeds, then this observation counts as a heroic expression of confidence. But if the plan fails miserably, then the tone of the quote might change retrospectively: A commander who admits that there is no backup plan but who baldly asserts that the mission will be successful seems reckless at best. This is not to suggest that Eisenhower was wrong to invade. But it is important to note that the judgment of the DDE depends a lot on how the issue is framed. If the invasion of Normandy had ultimately failed, we would not attribute bad intentions to the general. We might, however, care that a disastrous failure was a readily foreseen consequence. The fact that the variables all happened to work out in a favorable manner is hardly a basis for a sound and consistent moral principle.

Sometimes there are adverse consequences to judging individual decisions in isolation from a larger social context. Solitary actions might be morally good or at least neutral, but their cumulative effect could be bad. For example, in any particular instance of a doctor writing a prescription for opioids, both the agent's intention and the foreseeable outcome could be good. The patient is in pain, and the doctor intends only to relieve it. However, the cumulative effect of thousands of doctors writing these prescriptions has been a massive epidemic of opioid addiction. If we focus solely on isolated actions, then we fail to recognize how particular choices contribute to larger social problems. When we discount foreseeability in favor of intent, then we have no way of criticizing doctors who simply want to relieve pain. This is true even though addiction and abuse are clearly foreseeable possible outcomes. Even if an agent's intention is good, he could still be complicit with a foreseeable social harm that was caused by thousands of individual choices.

Sorting out questions of intention and causation is exceedingly complicated, and acknowledging this is nothing new. This recognition can be found in the corpus of the modern philosopher who was preoccupied with both concepts: Immanuel Kant. Although Kant is often portrayed as an absolutely certain deontologist, his writings demonstrate a remarkable amount of sensitivity and curiosity about intent and causation. It is easy to overlook this fact: His unequivocal condemnation of suicide presupposes a strict version of the DDE. While suicide is always morally prohibited, heroic sacrifice is always praiseworthy. This is because the agent has neither intended nor caused her own death. Kant even deems Cato's decision to kill himself rather than become Caesar's slave to be a cowardly and immoral act.[12] His action is self-caused, and he is solely responsible for it.

Elsewhere in his writings, however, Kant adopts a skeptical attitude toward our ability to determine intent and causation. In *Metaphysics of Morals*, Kant affirms a high standard for his philosophical project: "Moral cognition of oneself, which seeks to penetrate into the depths (the abyss) of one's heart which are quite difficult to fathom, is the beginning of all human wisdom."[13] Yet only a few paragraphs later, he claims, "The depths of the human heart are unfathomable. Who knows himself well enough to say, when he feels the incentive to fulfill his duty, whether it proceeds entirely from the representation of the law or whether there are not many other sensible impulses contributing to it that look to one's advantage (or to avoiding what is detrimental) and that, in other circumstances, could just as well serve vice?"[14]

It is not clear how one's own heart could be both "quite difficult to fathom" and "unfathomable." Nonetheless, Kant is adamant that morality involves some degree of self-knowledge, which in turn means understanding one's intentions. These intentions have causal efficacy in cases of suicide, where the outcome is both foreseen and intended. However, even if we put in the effort to understand our intentions, we are simply not good judges of our hearts. If we are too prone to pride and self-deception, then what is morally crucial might also be ultimately inscrutable.

The DDE attempts to solve this problem of inscrutability by simply *stipulating* that PAS must involve both foresight and intention. But claiming that this must be true based on the definition of suicide does nothing to help us understand the complex moral psychology of terminal cancer patients. Recall the example from the introduction of the hospice patient asking whether it was wrong to pray to die. The fact that he asked this question was evidence of a moral struggle, not a clearly identifiable intention. On the other hand, patients and doctors who participate in CSD have good intentions *by definition*. What they foresee and what they intend are, by fiat, two different things. Set aside Kant's concern about the inscrutability of one's own heart. An even more basic question is whether and by what right we can build an account of intentions and causation into the very definitions that we use to make sense of end-of-life dilemmas.

On Kant's view, intentions are both morally significant and (possibly) unfathomable. But this conflict can be resolved if we recognize that his analysis takes place on two different levels. From a theoretical perspective, a good intention is a necessary but not sufficient condition for a moral action. An action cannot be genuinely moral if it was not produced in the right way, but the fact that one has a good intention does not make whatever one does moral. The consequence must also be morally good. From a practical point of view, we cannot know whether any particular action has in fact been produced in this way. So Kant's view on this subject is not a decision procedure that helps us to sort out the intention of any particular agent. Rather, it is a meta-analysis of what it would mean for an action to be genuinely moral.

Our contemporary use of the DDE does not recognize this distinction. We assume that we can achieve in practice what we believe to be true theoretically: providing an adequate account of intention and causation in order to determine whether an action was moral. The DDE accomplishes this simply by stipulating that PAS and CSD are categorically distinct. As we have seen, there are many reasons to be suspicious of the ways in which we carve up reality in order to fit it into these two neat categories.

***

Assume for the sake of argument that every instance of PAS is a clear violation of the DDE and that every case of CSD obviously satisfies the relevant criteria. Even then, it would be wrong to apply the DDE to these end-of-life dilemmas.

An important feature of the DDE is the idea that whatever harm is imposed indirectly must be proportionate to (and not exceed) the good and intended outcome. As I mentioned earlier, one is justified in self-defense but only if the response is proportionate to the threat. But in the case of CSD, there is no way of knowing whether the harm imposed by deliberately inducing a permanent loss of consciousness is proportionate to the eradication of pain. It might seem intuitive to think that it is proportionate, but this assumption is not permitted by the idea of informed consent. In other words, we cannot simply speculate about what a patient might value.

I have already identified the problem of obtaining informed consent when continuous sedation is an inevitable outcome and not a genuine choice. I argued that this is especially true when patients are misleadingly told that they will suffer a loss of social interaction or merely subjective death. But another problem for this assumption is the fact that a patient can freely decline any medical treatment, even if it results in pain or death. This occurs when they are still able to give consent, such as a Jehovah's Witness refusing a blood transfusion or a cancer patient declining chemotherapy. So it is not good enough to simply assume that a permanent loss of consciousness must be a proportionate harm. And it is not sensible to ask a patient who is already experiencing intractable pain. What is required is some prior opportunity for the patient to determine whether this is acceptable. PAS provides this opportunity, this genuine choice, whereas CSD *on its own* does not.

Only the terminally ill patient is in any position to make a judgment about proportionate harm. Even if she judges her own permanent loss of consciousness to indeed be proportionate, she must do so as a consenting agent and not as "collateral damage." In other words, the doctrine of double effect is once again misapplied if it presupposes that the patient is in the same position as the civilian who happened to be near a high-value military target. The patient is, or should be, the central concern. Moreover, the permanent loss of consciousness is not an unintended and indirectly caused "side effect." The *whole point* of CSD is to relieve the patient of her capacity to experience the intractable pain. This is both intended and directly caused, whereas the loss of innocent life in war is neither intended nor directly caused.

This observation has been overlooked in debates over end-of-life sedation. Instead, the debates have been dominated by an easily answered empirical question: whether administering CSD speeds up the death of the organism. It does not, so long as the dosage is titrated properly.[15] If it were the case that a patient died from a pharmacological overdose, then that would be involuntary euthanasia, not CSD. A lack of nutrition and hydration might speed up the process, but we have deemed that to be a legitimate form of treatment refusal. On my view, the relevant concern is the intentional and directly caused eradication of consciousness.

So regardless of what one concludes about the possibility of determining intent and causation, the DDE is still misapplied in an important way to end-of-life dilemmas. We cannot ensure proportionality without a PAS alternative, something the DDE purports to forbid. Even if we could do this, the patient is, or should be, in a completely different position from the innocent bystander. Finally, inducing a permanent loss of consciousness cannot count as a side effect when it is the very point. Whether one prefers or rejects the higher brain model of death I discussed in the last chapter, intentionally causing its functional equivalent *for the patient* is a clear violation of the DDE.

There is one final problem with applying the DDE in this end-of-life context. As I mentioned earlier, some versions require that the action restore the status quo. This requirement is closely related to the proportionality criterion. Just as foreseeable but unintended harm cannot be excessive, it also cannot be imposed indefinitely. It is clear why this criterion would matter in the context of war. If a nation adequately defends itself but then decides to launch a preemptive attack, it is directly violating the DDE. But the founders of the Just War tradition obviously could not anticipate technological advances (e.g., drones) that would make indefinite war possible. Nor could they foresee the prevalence of new strategies (e.g., suicide bombing) that make it difficult, or even impossible, to restore the status quo.

The rise of drone warfare has made it much harder to determine whether the DDE has been satisfied. Any isolated action (e.g., bombing a weapons cache near a hospital) takes place in a new and complicated context. And the DDE seems designed to help us make one-off judgments, not to evaluate an entirely new age of warfare. Suppose that a drone strike on a terror camp kills a high-value target but also several other "men of combat age."[16] This singular event cannot be understood on its own. For instance, we would have to know how to define an enemy combatant to know how much collateral damage has been caused. This is difficult to determine when soldiers no longer wear uniforms, fly banners, and line up in rows.

We would also need to know counterfactually how much damage other strategies might have caused. If a drone strike is usually more precise than other methods, then we might sanction the collateral damage it causes. But none of these questions addresses the real issue: Do these new weapons create the conditions for permanent war? Are drones a pragmatic (and casualty-reducing) method of responding to the indefinite threat of terrorism? Or do they indirectly foster it?

Restoring the status quo is an important feature of the DDE in the context of war, but it is not clear how it could be applied in end-of-life dilemmas. Under normal conditions, medicine is designed to restore a status quo that has been disrupted by illness. But intentionally inducing a permanent loss of consciousness does not do this. There is no status quo left to restore. There are only hard choices about how to manage suffering and the process of dying. In his remarkable book *Being Mortal: Medicine and What Matters in the End*, Atul Gawande describes end-of-life dilemmas as a series of managed choices.[17] As a physician, he had a lot of experience guiding patients through this difficult process. But when his own father's health started to fail, the professional became personal. One difficult decision led to another and to another after that. For Dr. Gawande and his father, this was a time of hope and anxiety, determination and uncertainty.

In the simple observation that end-of-life dilemmas are really a series of managed choices, we discover the most subtle but damning objection to applying the DDE at the end of life. In contrast to the many concerns and contradictions discussed earlier, this flaw is more fundamental. Using the DDE in this context constitutes a kind of wish fulfillment. We are desperate for a moral principle to sanction the difficult decisions that we are forced to make. Any such principle would require that we isolate one particular choice in order to render a general verdict. Our principle is the DDE, and its object is the distinction between physician-assisted suicide and continuous sedation until death.

But just as warfare has evolved technologically and strategically, so has medicine: We are too good at dealing with pain and not good enough at curing disease. Unlike the death of an innocent bystander, a terminal cancer patient's death is both imminent and inevitable. In other words, the context for end-of-life dilemmas is not a freely chosen action (like bombing a terror camp), but an illness that we can neither prevent nor control.

For this reason, an end-of-life decision is better described as a "devil's choice." In his article, "The Devil's Choice: Re-Thinking Law, Ethics, and Symptom Relief in Palliative Care," Roger Magnusson explores the meaning of this phrase, using it as "a metaphor to describe medical choices that arise in circumstances where all the available options are both unwanted and perverse."[18] This is not to suggest that any decisions we could make would all be equally wrong. Rather, it means that no overarching principle (like the doctrine of double effect) can provide us with a single morally sanctioned outcome.

In this series of managed choices, all of our options are unwanted (i.e., death is imminent and inevitable) and perverse: Either a patient is permitted to self-administer a fatal dose, or she is compelled to consent to pharmacological oblivion. This is yet another reason, on my view, having a PAS option does not follow from having a right to die. Calling it a right would be to offer another general and decisive answer, another way of glossing over the specificity of a patient's dilemma. As Dr. Gawande discovered once end-of-life dilemmas became a personal issue, there is no escape. For a terminally ill patient, there are only unwanted and perverse options.

I close this chapter with a compelling example of a devil's choice. This story raised fascinating questions about sedation in the national media. In her book *Five Days at Memorial: Life and Death in a Storm-Ravaged Hospital*, Sheri Fink gives a startling account of the events that transpired at Memorial Hospital during Hurricane Katrina.[19] Dr. Anna Pou is the main character in this real-life drama. No one questions her bravery in staying to care for the many bed-bound patients; however, it was her method of caring for her patients that caused a moral uproar.

Dr. Pou assumed a position of authority and devised a novel triage system to evacuate the healthiest patients first. Further, she mandated that any patient with a Do Not Resuscitate order also be evaluated last. These two controversial decisions pale in comparison with what happened next. It was becoming increasingly evident that no one was coming to help the patients and staff stranded in the hospital. As the crisis wore on, they had to endure stifling heat, rising floodwaters, and a lack of electricity that rendered life-saving machines useless. In fact, the staff had to manually "bag" patients who could not breathe on their own, manually forcing air into their lungs. The psychological conditions are unfathomable: There were rampant rumors of looting, murders, and rapes. Many on the staff feared what might happen if such criminals, whether real or hypothetical, were to gain entry into the hospital. Even to call it a hospital seems strange, for it must have felt more like a war zone.

Dr. Pou judged that many bed-bound, untreated, and suffering patients were not candidates for evacuation. Even if outside help were to arrive on helicopters and boats, she thought it unlikely or even impossible that these patients would make it out alive. With the cooperation of some other members of the staff, she decided to inject at least seventeen of these patients with a cocktail of morphine and midazolam. None of these patients made it out alive.

After having been initially charged for her involvement in the deaths of these patients, the district attorney declined to prosecute. Dr. Pou never lost her medical license. Over the past decade, she has not only maintained her innocence, but she has also doubled-down on her controversial actions. She had advocated for new legislation that would certify that she made the right decisions. This includes legal protection for doctors and nurses from civil and criminal liability in times of crisis. It also includes the explicit approval of her triage method.

This case is an interesting test for the explanatory power of the DDE. Dr. Pou's criminal defense would have turned on the question of her intent and a determination of the cause of death. She has consistently maintained that her only intent was to relieve suffering. The conditions in the pseudo-hospital were so bad that relieving suffering required a heavy dose of pharmaceuticals. Dr. Pou would have had to explain why she administered both a heavy dose and a mixed cocktail that she should have known to suppress breathing. So the quantity and combination of the drugs found in the patients' systems would have been a key issue at trial. However, it would have been a serious challenge for a coroner to determine the toxicity of these drugs in corpses that were discovered a full ten days after the event. One coroner in particular was set to testify that any claims about drug toxicity as the cause of death would have been speculative at best.[20]

Let us set aside the question of determining a cause of death. The problem with valorizing intent is that one must then be able to describe another person's action as deliberate and its outcome as willed. Dr. Pou does not deny that she deliberately injected these patients with this drug cocktail. She does, however, deny that she willed their deaths as a direct outcome. She informally appealed to the DDE to make sense of this claim. Based on its logic, these deaths were a foreseeable but unintended consequence of her palliative efforts. Even if one could somehow prove that she intended that outcome, she would argue, in layman's terms, that she did not reflectively endorse the actions that she felt compelled to take. In fact, when pressed about the cause of death at trial, Dr. Pou would have argued that Hurricane Katrina killed those patients. Their conditions were terminal, even though many were not even that sick.

Dr. Pou and her staff faced a true devil's choice: administer a heavy and mixed dose of pharmaceuticals, foreseeing (and possibly even intending) that this would speed up their deaths. Or permit some degree of suffering in the short term, while anticipating extreme suffering and inevitable death in the event that the staff would be forced to evacuate without these patients.

The DDE does not help us to make any sense of this moral dilemma. Depending on how one construes Dr. Pou's intent, it can be used both to condemn and to defend her actions. But more importantly, it cannot offer us respite from the devil's choice. Even if she could foresee and intend these deaths, the alternative was no less unwanted or perverse. Even the medical staff that fled on boats and later criticized Dr. Pou are fully implicated here. You cannot escape responsibility by shirking your duty to stay. But if you stay, you have no good options.

I submit that the drama in Memorial Hospital is different in degree but not different in kind from ordinary end-of-life dilemmas. The DDE purports to sanction an absolute difference between physician-assisted suicide and continuous sedation until death. For the many reasons I have already discussed in this chapter, I do not accept the logic of this argument. But I think it is also worth noting that we crave a moral principle to absolve us from responsibility for making an unwanted and perverse choice. Unfortunately, wishing that this were real does not make it so.

NOTES

1. In fact, Eisenhower drafted a public message to deliver in case the invasion failed. Accessed August 6, 2016, https://www.archives.gov/education/lessons/d-day-message/images/failure-message.gif.

2. *Vacco v. Quill*, U.S. Supreme Court, 521 U.S. 793 (1997).

3. *Vacco v. Quill*.

4. Naimah Jabali-Nash, "Husband Sacrifices Life for Pregnant Wife in Crash, Occupants of Oncoming Car on Drugs, Say Cops," *CBS News*, September 13, 2010, accessed May 27, 2014, http://www.cbsnews.com/news/husband-sacrifices-life-for-pregnant-wife-in-crash-occupants-of-oncoming-car-on-drugs-say-cops/.

5. In chapter 9 of their book, Leo Kahane and Stephen Shmanske attempt to quantify bloodlust among hockey fans. Motocross and NASCAR would serve as suitable examples, too. See Kahane and Shmanske, *The Oxford Handbook of Sports Economics: Volume 1: The Economics of Sports* (Oxford: Oxford University Press, 2012).

6. This data comes from the nation's largest brain bank. It was reported across multiple news outlets, but the best summary can be found at Jason Bellow, "New: 87 Deceased NFL Players Test Positive for Brain Disease," *Frontline*, September 18, 2015, accessed June 1, 2016, http://www.pbs.org/wgbh/frontline/article/new-87-deceased-nfl-players-test-positive-for-brain-disease/.

7. See Dave Philipps, "Suicide Rate among Veterans Has Risen Sharply since 2001," *New York Times*, July 7, 2016, accessed August 13, 2016, http://www.nytimes.com/2016/07/08/us/suicide-rate-among-veterans-has-risen-sharply-since-2001.html?_r=0.

8. See especially Will Kymlicka, *Liberalism, Community, and Culture* (Oxford: Clarendon, 1989), and Ronald Dworkin, *Sovereign Virtue: The Theory and Practice of Equality* (Cambridge, MA: Harvard University Press, 2000), 216-218. The literature on this topic is extensive, and the disagreements run deep. It is outside the scope of this book to give a thorough account of the debates in autonomy theory. Here I am appealing to the most basic version of the endorsement constraint as intuitively plausible, even if it turns out to have some philosophical flaws when fully fleshed out. In other words, I think it fits our folk psychological beliefs about what it could mean to deliberately do something that we do not genuinely intend. My examples reflect this.

9. Tom Junod, "The Falling Man," *Esquire Magazine*, September 2003, accessed November 12, 2015, http://classic.esquire.com/the-falling-man/. This essay inspired an interesting film by the same name.

10. See the short entry on Rommel in PBS, "American Experience: D-Day," accessed December 5, 2014, http://www.pbs.org/wgbh/amex/dday/peopleevents/p_rommel.html.

11. The National World War II Museum has published an exquisitely detailed account of the D-Day invasion, accessed February 6, 2015, http://www.nationalww2museum.org/learn/education/for-students/ww2-history/d-day-june-6-1944.html.

12. See Immanuel Kant, *Lectures on Ethics*, ed. and trans. Peter Heath (Cambridge: Cambridge University Press, 1997), 144-49.

13. Immanuel Kant, *Metaphysics of Morals*, in *Practical Philosophy*, trans. Mary Gregor (Cambridge: Cambridge University Press, 1996), 6:441.

14. Kant, *Metaphysics of Morals*, 447.

15. See especially Nigel Sykes and Andrew Thorns, "The Use of Opioids and Sedatives at the End of Life," *Lancet Oncology* 1 (2003): 312–18.

16. The way in which deaths by drone strikes get counted is a persistent source of speculation. Some critics allege that the CIA secretly fudges the data by counting all "men of combat age" as legitimate terror targets. Others either deny that this happens or defend this method of distinguishing legitimate targets from collateral damage. See Jo Becker and Scott Shane, "Secret 'Kill List' Proves a Test of Obama's Principles and Will," *New Yoirk Times*, May 29, 2012, accessed June 2, 2014, http://www.nytimes.com/2012/05/29/world/obamas-leadership-in-war-on-al-qaeda.html.

17. Atul Gawande, *Being Mortal: Medicine and What Matters in the End* (New York: Metropolitan Books, 2014).

18. This quote comes from the abstract of Roger S. Magnusson, "The Devil's Choice: Re-Thinking Law, Ethics, and Symptom Relief in Palliative Care," *Journal of Law, Medicine, and Ethics* 34, no. 3 (Fall 2006): 559-69.

19. Sheri Fink, *Five Days at Memorial: Life and Death in a Storm-Ravaged Hospital* (New York: Broadway Books, 2016).

20. Fink, *Five Days at Memorial*, 257. On p. 394, Fink reports that the American Medical Association was *at the very same time* considering the proposal that they later adopted in 2008: ethical approval of continuous sedation until death for otherwise intractable pain.

Chapter Four

On Suicide, Acceptance, and Control

Visitors to the French Quarter in New Orleans have a dizzying array of options to while away an afternoon. Many of them (though certainly not all) involve learning something about the past. It would be both impossible and beside the point to separate fact from fiction in the voodoo tales of Marie Leveau or the pirate narratives of Jean Lafitte. Sometimes it is simply better to be captivated by a good story.

However, there is a little gem of a museum tucked away on Chartres Street where one can absorb some real and important history. It is only a mile away from the World War II Museum, where one can study the circumstances of a fascinating example of the doctrine of double effect. It is less than four miles from the old Memorial Hospital, where Dr. Pou terminally sedated (or euthanized) patients during Hurricane Katrina. The New Orleans Pharmacy Museum is a treasure trove of old artifacts and information. If you arrive in time for the 1:00 p.m. tour, you will get more than a good story. The history of pharmaceuticals in America is perhaps the most amusing and deadly serious account one would care to hear on a weekday afternoon.

As the causes of various terrible diseases were being debated in the early and middle nineteenth century, so, too, were some possible remedies. Anyone could weigh in on this subject! There were no pharmaceutical regulations (or at least none that were ever enforced) prior to 1804. At that time, a three-hour qualifying oral exam was established, and Louis Dufilho later became American's first licensed pharmacist in 1816.[1] Interestingly, the New Orleans Pharmacy Museum is located in Dufilho's old apothecary. This formal process was hardly a rigorous accreditation, but it was the start of something new.

In the middle and even late nineteenth century, the ancient miasma theory continued to compete with modern germ theory, as promulgated by Louis

Pasteur and his colleagues. Firing cannons into the swamp and burning tar were two ways to disturb the "bad air" that supposedly caused incurable illnesses like smallpox, cholera, and yellow fever. Pasteur, the founder of microbiology, ultimately put these pseudoremedies to rest and ushered in a new era of vaccines.

This major advancement in modern medicine, coupled with the birth of pharmacy as a recognized profession earlier in the century, produced profound changes in the treatment of disease. For the first time ever, there was both a correct consensus on the cause of disease and an officially recognized profession for relieving its symptoms. Competing theories of disease and quacks peddling placebos were soundly defeated (though, to be sure, quacks never completely go away).

The consolidation of medical and pharmaceutical authority continued into the twentieth century. The 1914 Harrison Act controlled and taxed the manufacture and distribution of opium and opium derivatives for the first time in American history.[2] This included, among other substances, morphine and heroin. The Harrison Act was later supplemented by legislation that regulated the medical use of these substances and criminalized their non-medical use. Its champion was William Jennings Bryan, who would later act as an outspoken advocate of Prohibition and an influential critic of evolution.

This was undoubtedly a decisive moment in the history of pharmaceutical regulation and control. Some might even argue that it was the beginning of the modern war on drugs. The 1970 Controlled Substances Act is the grandson of the Harrison Act. It empowered the federal government to determine which substances qualified for Schedule I status, the strictest form of regulation.

In the last chapter, I raised some questions concerning the application of the doctrine of double effect to end-of-life dilemmas. I focused especially on the epistemological problems associated with determining intent, causation, and proportionate harm. In this chapter, I discuss the topics of acceptance and control that are found throughout the literature on physician-assisted suicide. Critics of PAS often claim that it transgresses a moral boundary between what human beings ought to determine (e.g., fighting disease) and what they should not (e.g., the manner and timing of death). I argue that these criticisms ignore the profound amount of control that has already been allocated to doctors and proxies in the century since the Harrison Act was passed. In a special way, offering specific patients a PAS option reclaims some authority for the individual patient in an era when much of it has been subtly, even imperceptibly, surrendered. Then I address a criticism of my view that suggests that both patients and doctors would undergo a kind of existential crisis if physician-assisted suicide were permitted.

There are two primary ways to defend PAS against the objection that it involves an unnatural and immoral amount of control over one's fate. One could concede that it does increase control in general while defending this as morally permissible. Or one could show how the control that one asserts through PAS is hardly unique to this action. PAS recoups a modicum of control for the patient that already exists for doctors and proxy decision makers. It should be permissible in specific cases by virtue of the fact that it redistributes control in morally appropriate ways. So while I am sympathetic to the first strategy, I focus on the second one.

It is difficult to address this objection concerning control, largely because of the terminology that has evolved to distinguish physician-assisted suicide from continuous sedation until death. On my view, this is yet another case of language causing confusion, of vocabulary obscuring ethical insight. This confusion goes at least as far back as the Hippocratic Oath, where modern ethics is born under the injunction to "first do no harm." Nonmaleficence claims a special ethical priority, and beneficence is only permissible once one has ruled out the possibility of harm. This fundamental distinction makes modern medical ethics duly risk averse: While the medical urge is to heal and restore, the basic ethical impulse is negative in nature. This produces certain psychological dispositions (i.e., being active or passive, controlling or accepting), as well as epistemological claims about a given decision (e.g., whether it is better described as an act or as an omission).

As we have already seen, the doctrine of double effect inherits the preoccupation with activity and passivity. Any harm must be only passively, as in indirectly and unintentionally, imposed. Intent is by definition an active desire as opposed to something that an agent could also passively will. So a terminally ill patient who self-administers a fatal dose of barbiturates is committing suicide, even if she desperately wants to live. Someone who routinely risks his life and confesses that he does not mind doing so is not suicidal. We can attribute only a high degree of foreseeability, not an active intention to die. Even if his reckless behavior were to result in his death, he would have only indirectly caused it.

Using this terminology, the difference between PAS and CSD is supposed to be clear. One death is actively intended and caused, while the other is indirectly produced through an omission (i.e., the withdrawal of medicine, nutrition, and hydration). However, on my view, continuous sedation until death must be evaluated as a separate action that is distinct from the patient's decision to refuse treatment. As I have already argued, informed consent is not sufficiently obtained under these conditions. And the death of the patient is *at the very least* passively willed, unlike any other example where the collateral damage is immediately and totally regretted. Suppose for a moment that a patient (or at least her organism) could magically continue to live for a decade in a persistent vegetative state even after all treatment is stopped. If the doctor or proxy had no intention whatsoever, either actively or passively, that the patient die, then they would have to approve of this senseless outcome or at least find it to be morally neutral.

It is misleading to suggest that "letting die" should count simply as an omission: It mixes the active decision of a patient or proxy, the doctor's adherence to that choice, the withdrawal of food and water, and the administering of superpharmaceuticals to permanently eradicate consciousness. According to the proponents of the higher-brain model of death, this last decision intentionally and directly causes the death of the patient.

Once we overcome a naive insistence that actions are categorically different from omissions, especially in situations where they are mixed together, we encounter another suspicious moral argument. Perhaps the key distinction is not between acts and omissions but between extraordinary and ordinary forms of treatment. This move has the merit of recognizing that we are discussing active choices at the end of life. It cautions, however, that extraordinary interventions are not required and can sometimes be immoral.

The 1975 *Quinlan* case established such a precedent, and it also made the public aware of the importance of advanced directives. When Karen Ann Quinlan slipped into a coma, doctors refused to comply with the wishes of the adoptive parents to take her off of a ventilator. The Supreme Court of Missouri ultimately ruled that a proxy could make this decision.[3] The appropriate standard of evidence was later clarified by the U.S. Supreme Court in the 1990 *Cruzan* case: A proxy must present clear and convincing evidence of a patient's intent.[4]

It is ironic that two of the main "treatment refusal cases, *Quinlan* and *Cruzan*,[5] both concern patients *who were already in a persistent vegetative state.* The absolute right to refuse treatment is supposed to guarantee bodily autonomy and prevent forced medication. But in these cases, and in countless others, the situation had already progressed past the point in which the patient could invoke this right for herself. So perhaps the right to refuse treatment is not a sufficient guarantor of patient consent after all.

Aside from this problem, we would still have to determine the difference between extraordinary and ordinary interventions. In the *Quinlan* case, the adoptive parents achieved their goal of removing Ms. Quinlan from the ventilator. They did not, however, believe that the feeding tube could count as an extraordinary measure. So Ms. Quinlan, or her organism, remained in a persistent vegetative state for *ten* more years, until her death in 1985. It is simply not plausible to believe that a ventilator counts as an extraordinary intervention, whereas a feeding tube does not. One instrument is larger and more complex than the other, but that hardly seems morally relevant. Introducing yet another distinction between natural and artificial forms of treatment would not help either. A ventilator and a feeding tube are both medical devices that maintain the life of an organism when it can no longer function properly. They are both scientific attempts to control natural processes that have broken down.

The U.S. Supreme Court should be commended for its affirmation of a strict standard of evidence for determining a patient's intent. However, we should also take note of the massive amount of control that doctors and proxies have in these situations. The fact that the standard of evidence is so high can actually be detrimental to a patient's goals, especially if there is no advance directive or if it is vague and open to interpretation. If a patient is already in a persistent vegetative state, then the default position is the view of the doctor and the proxy. Clear and convincing evidence would be required to establish the unconscious (or dead) patient's view. This is hard to come by and impossible in many cases.

As there was no such evidence in the *Quinlan* case, we will never know whether Ms. Quinlan would have agreed with the idiosyncratic and morally suspicious claim that a ventilator and a feeding tube are categorically different forms of treatment. So we could never know if she would have approved of letting her organism live on for another ten years. Nor could we know if she would have endorsed the doctor's view that removing a patient from a feeding tube would count as homicide. All we have are two competing and equally implausible accounts coming from sources *other* than Ms. Quinlan herself.

In the cases of Ms. Quinlan and Ms. Cruzan, catastrophic damage had already occurred. They were obviously not candidates for physician-assisted suicide since they were already permanently unconscious. However, on my view, the control that a patient wishes to exert over her condition when she requests a fatal dose of barbiturates is not a unique form of control. And the fact that she self-administers the dose rather than having misguided spokespersons arguing on her behalf is morally significant.

We try to carve up end-of-life dilemmas in terms of acts and omissions, extraordinary and ordinary interventions, and even natural and artificial remedies. But in doing so, we isolate particular elements of the dilemma and ignore the context that makes them intelligible. We forget that each event is a complicated and interrelated mix of elements, and we willfully ignore our own motivations to deny that we actively, extraordinarily, or artificially cause a death.

***

In addition to doctor and proxy control in specific cases, we should notice that the evolution of superpharmaceuticals has *radically* increased control over the manner and timing of death in general. Yet our discussions of sedation at the end of life have been ripped from the history and context that make them significant. There are many possible uses of the kinds of superpharmaceuticals at issue in end-of-life debates. They are used recreationally, during surgery, on death row, in hospitals, and in hospices. The development of (and carefully circumscribed control over) barbiturates, anesthetics, opioids, and sedatives are not morally neutral facts. Rather, these drugs have serious implications for the kind of power and authority that some individuals can exercise over others.

Sometimes the use and abuse of these drugs makes headlines. The death of the beloved comedian Chris Farley in 1997 reminded us that morphine could be involved in an accidental overdose. In 2013, Missouri decided not to use Propofol in lethal injections. This was partly due to public outcry after Conrad Murray (the smoothest of criminals) used this drug to sedate the King of Pop to death four years earlier.[6]

For the most part, though, these drugs are used privately and behind closed doors: in hospitals, hospices, nursing homes, and prisons. So it is unconvincing to claim *by fiat* that medical providers fulfill the conditions of the doctrine of double effect when they use these drugs for palliation. We would have to analyze intention and causality in any particular case in order to say anything about it. Likewise, it is a mistake to simply assert that using these drugs for the purpose of lethal injection must be a more humane form of death in comparison to other, more medieval methods. In both cases, we make the mistake of automatically deferring to what is done by the relevant authorities away from public scrutiny.

We discovered this recently when the European Union embargo on lethal injection drugs, like sodium thiopental, dried up supply in the United States. This has forced states to experiment with different drug cocktails, with uniformly disastrous results.[7] Ohio, for instance, has used a two-drug cocktail of midazolam and hydromorphone, a morphine derivative. Interestingly, this mixture mimicked the combination used by Dr. Pou in Memorial Hospital. In this case, however, the cocktail caused profound suffering. Ohio is not alone in inflicting this new form of suffering on its prisoners.[8]

The situation has gotten so desperate that the FDA had to confiscate illegal shipments of sodium thiopental that were bound for Arizona and Texas.[9] Compounding the problem is that doctors are not usually permitted to mix these drugs since it violates their ethical code.[10] In response to this new problem, Utah legalized the use of the firing squad, claiming that it would be a more humane form of death. A prisoner could be killed instantly by an expert marksman instead of suffering excruciatingly from air hunger for over twenty minutes.

It is possible that the European Union embargo could indirectly end the death penalty in the United States. If lethal injection cannot fulfill its original purpose (a more humane form of death), then the entire practice could be permanently discarded.

There is no such scrutiny surrounding the administration of the same categories of drugs for the purpose of continuous sedation until death. Permanently eradicating the consciousness of a terminally ill patient is seen as a morally and medically necessary alternative to physician-assisted suicide. But what is it about the new lethal injection crisis that makes it morally wrong? On one view, it is the violation of the injunction against cruel and unusual punishment. More forceful critics of the death penalty would have a broader argument against the authority of the state to kill its citizens. The fact that the prisoner suffers immensely is a way of capturing the public imagination, but it is not the main reason the action is wrong. Similarly, the fact that CSD offers a peaceful pharmacological oblivion should not blind us to the fact that it also grants immense power to doctors and proxies.

Exclusive control over superpharmaceuticals has been allocated to doctors and pharmacists for the past century. The regulation of these industries in the nineteenth and twentieth centuries is obviously a sign of progress. Yet it seems a little disingenuous to disavow the power that one possesses, especially after obtaining exclusive authority over these drugs.

The scientific authority of continuous sedation until death depends upon the assertion that death and medicine are to be defined relative to the status of an organism. I have already discussed many reasons this assertion is unfounded or at least insufficiently defended. We grant doctors the authority to determine death because we assume that they must be experts at it, even though it is a conceptual (and not simply empirical) question. I have also argued that, in the case of diagnosing death, we often fall victim to a "false sense of scientific objectivity." CSD is yet another source of authority and control in end-of-life dilemmas.

But now notice how the doctrine of double effect works hand in glove with these scientific assertions. For instance, it corroborates the assumption that death involves the killing of an organism. And even if the permanent loss of consciousness is a form of collateral damage, it is simply assumed to be a proportionate form of harm. So ethicists affirm the authority of doctors and proxies, who then deny that they actively control the manner and timing of a patient's death. They assert this without also explicitly defending the supreme moral significance of the brain stem.

The DDE, then, gives us a "false sense of ethical objectivity." It purports to provide us with a critical understanding of end-of-life dilemmas, when it simply rubber-stamps preexisting assumptions. This ethical principle models and mirrors the supposedly scientific principle that defines death as the total loss of brain function. Instead of challenging physiological assumptions, it uncritically adopts them.

We exert control up to *and including* the moment in which a patient is continuously sedated. We do so by actively administering the dose of morphine and by intentionally and directing causing the permanent loss of consciousness. All of this occurs against the backdrop of a drama two centuries in the making: the consolidation of power for doctors and pharmacists. And all of this is ethically sanctioned by a principle that concedes rather than challenges our suspicious physiological presuppositions.

On my view, PAS simply redistributes the authority and control that already exists but that is now allocated to doctors and proxies. It is morally preferable to allow the patient herself to have the final say, provided that she can competently choose to self-administer the fatal dose. The clear and convincing standard of evidence is seen as strict but only with reference to other standards that permit testimony, like hearsay. If the patient is available to actively consent, then this is the clearest and most convincing evidence one could ask for.

Carving a PAS exception for terminally ill patients is an honest recognition that CSD is, for the patient herself, functionally equivalent to death. Regardless of how one wishes to define death for the purpose of public policy, inducing permanent unconsciousness means that the person will no longer be around to experience anything at all. Physician-assisted suicide was not an available remedy for Ms. Quinlan or Ms. Cruzan. But it could be for patients who are terminally ill and conscious of that fact.

These patients have the same hope for a peaceful death as someone who would consent to her organism outliving her person. They do not, however, have access to the means by which this could be achieved. That option has been foreclosed to them, at least in an official and legally recognized way, over the course of the past century. So the professionals who have been granted the legal and ethical authority to control the manufacture and distribution of superpharmaceuticals should not view themselves as merely passive purveyors of pain relief.

Finally, it rings hollow to suggest that terminally ill patients who request access to these drugs are trying to control their fate. There is no generalizable attitude that we could ascribe to these patients. But if there were, it would likely be an attitude of acceptance rather than control. As modest as we make continuous sedation sound, it forbids the killing of a cancer-ridden organism, even as it deliberately terminates the person. For a patient requesting PAS under these conditions, this might seem like an extreme imposition and an obvious exercise in control.

I have already argued that a patient could reasonably prefer that her person and organism die simultaneously. Now suppose that she accepts her fate and resents the control that CSD would exert over her end-of-life prospects. Here again we run up against the limits of language: To say that she has accepted her fate might connote a sense of sad resignation. On this view, PAS would be a small consolation, a final attempt to wrest control over nature. But acceptance need not mean passive resignation nor provide the impetus for active and illicit control in the form of physician-assisted suicide.

The patient might find some freedom and satisfaction in the prospect of self-administering the fatal dose. There is some evidence that merely having this as an option achieves this effect.[11] All things being equal, she desperately wants to live. But she understands that things are never equal in this way. She approaches her mortality with a sense of equanimity, a calmness that should not be mistaken for sad and simple resignation.

There might not be a word that adequately conveys the patient's attitude in this case. I think that the German word *Versöhnung* comes closest to expressing this sentiment. This word translates as "reconciliation," but its meaning is more nuanced than that. Michael Hardimon writes of the complex nature of this kind of reconciliation as follows: "In contrast to 'reconciliation,' *Versöhnung* strongly connotes a process of transformation. When two parties become genuinely *versöhnt*, they do not resume their old relationship unchanged. They become *versöhnt* by changing their behavior and attitudes in fundamental ways. Parties who have attained *Versöhnung* do not have to decide to get along together; their getting along together is, instead, the natural result of their being in a new, transformed state."[12]

A terminally ill patient who requests PAS might be reconciled to her condition in just this way. The kind of transformation that Hardimon describes involves neither active control nor passive acceptance. It is also not entirely cognitive since it was not brought about by a decision or simply willed into existence. It might be described as a Stoic form of acceptance or as a form of freedom that does not depend upon changing what will occur. As Gregory Hays puts it, "The Stoics [defined] free will as a voluntary accommodation to what is in any case inevitable. According to this theory, man is like a dog tied to a moving wagon. If the dog refuses to run along with the wagon he will be dragged by it, yet the choice remains his: to run or be dragged."[13]

It is understandable, even common, to find some Stoic analogies a little disturbing. The examples they used were designed to shock the sensibilities of the reader.[14] So comparing a terminally ill patient to a dog tied to a moving wagon might seem inelegant. However, it aptly describes the patient's situation, as well as the only sense of freedom she will ever know.

The Stoics were compatibilists on the question of free will. In other words, they believed that we are free to conform our judgments to an already-determined external reality. We are not free in the sense of being able to change that reality as we see fit. Whether this account is true in general or not, it is the exact situation in which the terminally ill patient finds herself. She is free only in the sense of adopting an attitude about her condition, not in changing what will happen to her. Which end-of-life option, PAS or CSD, is more like being dragged by the moving wagon, and which resembles voluntarily running behind it?

Referencing a Stoic form of freedom is not *at all* to romanticize the decision to self-administer a fatal dose. I have already described such a decision as a devil's choice, where every option is unwanted or perverse. It is, however, to suggest that the distinction between acceptance and control is a red herring. It is closer to the truth to suggest that the transformation some terminally ill patients might experience is a complicated mix of both attitudes. The prohibition of a PAS option is more straightforward, as it imposes uniformity on a psychologically and morally complex situation. This is not because such a prohibition violates some purported right to die. Rather, it is because the patient is rendered a passive recipient of medical care without having provided adequate informed consent.

***

This affirmation of Stoic freedom will strike critics of PAS as an insufficient basis for public policy. Even if there were some commendable end-of-life attitude that could make PAS legitimate, this would not show that a general right to die should be established. On this point, I absolutely agree. My defense of PAS has taken the form of a carefully carved exception, not a general right to die. However, I think that attempts to dismiss any PAS claim as a merely subjective preference are morally suspicious. We saw one such effort earlier, when Daniel Callahan argued that "idiosyncratic" preferences, including access to PAS, could not form the basis of public policy. Nor could a subjective preference to die ever trump an inalienable right to life. However, these preferences are not idiosyncratic and inscrutable, even if they are personal.[15] They are also rationally intelligible.

A more sensitive and refined defense of Callahan's view is presented by J. David Velleman in an article titled "Against the Right to Die." Velleman immediately grants that any particular person expressing a desire to die might be morally entitled to assistance.[16] He opposes, however, an institutional right to die. (Note: He discusses euthanasia rather than PAS specifically, so I use the phrase "assisted death" in this context.)

Velleman's main concern is that even *presenting* death as an option to some patients could count as a subtle form of coercion. So it is out of respect for patients, and not in an attempt to control their choices, that assisted death is better left out of the range of options. He writes, "Offering someone an alternative to the status quo makes two outcomes possible for him, but neither of them is the outcome that was possible before. He can now choose the status quo or choose the alternative, but he can no longer *have* the status quo without *choosing* it."[17] In other words, when continued existence is not simply assumed as a default position, then a patient "will rightly be perceived as the agent of his own survival."[18]

On this view, forcing a choice between assisted death and continued existence would put a tremendous burden on some patients. They would be more prone to manipulation by their family or even by society at large. Velleman notes that we do not exactly value the lives of the ill and infirm. He worries that this social pressure would only escalate once a patient becomes incapable of "independent activity" and is more dependent on others.[19] If she is forced to justify her continued existence but finds that she lacks good reasons, then assisted death becomes more than a morally neutral option. Instead, it becomes a suggestion.

This view is commendable for its even-handed approach to this difficult topic. It is sensible to claim that simply having death as an option could prompt a patient to formulate reasons to live or die. When this option is presented by an authority figure and reiterated by a family member, then this pressure could increase. However, there are many interesting problems with Velleman's approach to the idea of assisted death. First, it ignores the fact that patient consent is *already* supposed to obtain in cases of CSD. In other words, the patient is not supposed to be a passive recipient of medical treatment. So to imply that choosing assisted death is categorically different from consenting to CSD is to admit that patients are not now, in fact, at the center of end-of-life dilemmas. Rather, doctors and proxies exert tremendous control over them. As I have argued at length, this does not sufficiently guarantee informed consent.

Second, Velleman seriously overstates the existential implications of having a PAS option. The notion that this option could create a kind of "paradox of choice"[20] is extremely far-fetched. It is true that having more rather than fewer options can sometimes mitigate rather than enhance one's freedom. For instance, strolling down a cereal aisle in a grocery store without having any prior sense of what to buy might result in temporary paralysis. Having to make an unguided choice between one hundred different options might even result in an irrational and regrettable purchase. Suppose that I choose the cereal with the brightest box or the goofiest mascot. This would be a baseless way of breaking the tie, and I could not claim that my choice was grounded in good reasons.

But why should we believe that having the option of assisted death would result in a similar paradox of choice? In contrast to any other example of this concept, there is an intuitive and immediate bias against dying. And this is especially true when we would be the cause of our own demise. In the following passage, Velleman discusses the very existential attitude upon which his thesis depends: "Now, the idea of surviving by default will be anathema to existentialists, who will insist that the choice between life and death is a choice that we have to make every day, perhaps every moment. Yet even if there is a deep, philosophical sense in which we do continually choose to go on living, it is not reflected in our ordinary self-understanding."[21]

This is exactly correct. So the burden falls squarely on the *opponent* of assisted death to explain how the mere option to die would induce an existential crisis. For someone unaccustomed to thinking of her continued existence as a choice, this will likely not even be a live "option" in any real sense. To put the point trivially, it would be more like a health-obsessed Grape Nuts addict walking down the grocery aisle and never being enticed by the ninety-nine other brands.

Further, the comprehensive American Medical Association study cited in chapter 1 provides us with some intriguing data on the question of patient anxiety: "In general, the existing evidence does not support the commonly held belief that communication about goals of care and end-of-life issues increases patient anxiety, depression, and/or hopelessness. Patients and families want open and honest information and a balance between realistic information and appropriate hope."[22] If a PAS option were honestly discussed in the context of a patient's end-of-life dilemma, then we would need a special reason (and perhaps some evidence, too) that it would cause a unique form of harm.

After making this remark about a hypothetical patient's existential attitude, Velleman wisely shifts his discussion from a patient who has options to a patient who is *perceived* to have them. In other words, even if assisted death is not a live option for the patient, it could become one if she feels pressure to respond to the perception of choice. It is not clear who or what is doing the perceiving in this case. Sometimes it seems like the family tacitly exerts pressure on the patient; other times the pressure takes the form of a social norm that views the lives of the ill and infirm as less valuable.

But is it fair to conflate a general attitude of discrimination with a disregard for whether the targets of this attitude live or die? We have been offered no reason to believe that this social norm could be translated into something absolutely more sinister. Nor do we have any reason to assume that the patient's doctor or family would tacitly exert pressure on her to opt for assisted death. There is insufficient evidence to establish this, so at best it is a speculative assumption. However, some evidence suggests that, on the contrary, people have quite different attitudes when considering their own mortality and when thinking about others. This includes both patients and loved ones![23] We tend to want more freedom and control for ourselves but more aggressive treatment for others. If this is so, then assumptions about social pressure fail in the same way as assumptions about a patient's own existential crisis.

Perhaps these attitudes would change if PAS becomes *widely* accepted or even approved of. In their article "Killing the Pain Not the Patient: Palliative Care vs. Assisted Suicide," Richard Doerflinger and Carlos Gomez write:

> Once the "quick and easy" solution of assisted suicide is accepted in a society, doctors lose the incentive to pursue more difficult but life-affirming ways of truly caring for patients close to death. The converse is also true: prohibiting assisted suicide sets a clear limit to doctors' options so they can commit themselves to the challenges of accompanying patients through their last days. As one physician said after years practicing hospice medicine: "Only because I

> knew that I could not and would not kill my patients was I able to enter most fully and intimately into caring for them as they lay dying."[24]

There are two separate but related claims here: The first concerns the general psychological state of doctors, while the second deals with its effect on the patient. This testimony from an anonymous physician asserts that PAS would undermine the patient–doctor relationship. We are asked to believe that doctors would no longer care for patients in the same way if a PAS "shortcut" were available to them. But this testimony seems terribly unconvincing. It is possibly true (but unverifiable) only for the particular doctor making this claim. When the doctor says that it was "*only because*" he knew that he "could not and would not" kill patients, what are we to make of this? Are we to believe that it is simply the force of law that prevents him from doing so? We are asked to believe that, if PAS were suddenly made legal, our anonymous physician's attitude would change, too. However, nonmaleficence is at the heart of medical practice. Every medical impulse and intuition rejects the idea of "killing" a patient. So why should we believe that physicians will embrace PAS just because it becomes permissible?

Frankly it is a little disturbing to learn that an experienced hospice physician would think this way. She already has all the tools necessary to speed up the process of death. A carefully titrated dose of morphine does not cause the death of the organism. But a hospice professional already controls the degree to which a patient is conscious. She could also illicitly overdose a patient. If the only thing preventing her from doing so is knowing that it would be illegal, then we should indeed be worried about the state of hospice care. This is especially true when the rigorous process of obtaining a fatal dose of barbiturates is frivolously described as a "quick and easy" solution.

The second claim in the citation is equally unnerving. One of the effects of the doctor's new psychological disposition would be to further undermine palliative care. This assertion can be paired with the idea that we will no longer attempt to medically treat depression. We are asked to believe that palliation will seem pointless and requires too much effort. The same goes for administering depression medication and monitoring mental health symptoms. So if PAS were permissible, then doctors would fail to provide adequate care. Instead, they would pursue assisted death as a shortcut.

Part of the problem is that critics of PAS cannot seem to get their story straight. Take, for instance, the observations of the New York Task Force on Life and the Law. Their influential report "When Death Is Sought—Assisted Suicide and Euthanasia in the Medical Context" rejects the legalization of PAS. The committee presents many of the typical arguments against physician-assisted suicide. Since this report was cited in the two majors PAS cases heard by the Supreme Court, it matters whether these arguments are presented in a clear and coherent fashion.

Before we examine the arguments, let us quickly note how misleading the title of the report really is. Patients who wish to self-administer a fatal dose of barbiturates are “seeking” death in the same way that those who jumped from the Twin Towers on 9/11 sought it. They have concluded that this part of the devil’s choice is better than the alternative. All things being equal, the vast majority of these patients probably wish that they were not afflicted with terminal cancer.

The authors are especially concerned about the stigma associated with sedating patients. They worry about patients being undermedicated, both in terms of pain relief and depression, and they are concerned that the debate over PAS exacerbates this problem. On their view, those who defend PAS by criticizing end-of-life sedation could stigmatize sedation and inadvertently cause needless suffering.

The question of the relationship between assisted death and palliation must be taken seriously and dealt with in a sensitive manner. However, the authors end up having to make contradicting arguments about the prevalence of this problem of patients being undermedicated. First, the authors claim that “depression is distinct from the normal feelings of sadness generally experienced by terminally ill patients. It is a myth that major clinical depression ordinarily accompanies terminal illness.”[25] But just two bullet points down in their list of objections, we are told that “uncontrolled pain, particularly when accompanied by feelings of hopelessness and untreated depression, is a significant contributing factor for suicide and suicidal ideation. Medications and pain relief techniques now make it possible to treat pain effectively for most patients.”[26] And in their very next observation, we learn that, “despite the fact that effective treatments are available, severely and terminally ill patients generally do not receive adequate relief from pain.”[27]

So major depression does not normally accompany terminal illness, but when left untreated, pain and untreated depression are significant contributing factors for suicide. This could mean that suicidal ideation is rare since major depression for terminally ill patients is a myth. In this case, PAS would not pose a threat to patients. As in the response to Velleman’s argument, physician-assisted suicide would not seem like a live option to most patients.

On the other hand, it could mean that doctors are reluctant to provide pain relief and that this leads to a serious problem of suicidal ideation. If this is true, then a patient might opt for assisted death just because she is experiencing physiological and psychological pain. But then legalizing PAS would make it *more* likely that doctors would adequately treat pain. If doctors are reluctant to cause harm to patients by overmedicating, then palliation will become *more* legitimate if PAS is an option.

Suppose that many doctors are presently concerned about causing harm by overmedicating. So their default option is to exercise caution and undertreat symptoms. If PAS were permissible, then the default option would still be nonmaleficence. But in this case, doctors would be reluctant to assist in a patient's death and more likely to adequately treat their symptoms. In other words, the reluctance to harm a patient by overmedicating would be rendered moot by the competing option: assisting in a suicide.

I think that this account of the psychology of doctors is far more compelling than the version we get in the comment from Doerflinger and Gomez. Perhaps we cannot really say anything in general about this issue. But if we can, I am confident in the claim that nonmaleficence is a basic medical impulse and intuition. If this is so, then it is unconvincing to argue that the prohibition on PAS is the only thing keeping doctors from killing patients. Further, it seems reasonable to suggest that a PAS option would remove the perceived risk of overmedicating patients. It would likely *reframe* for doctors what counts as a risky option in the first place.

There is one final view to consider before we leave this line of argument. Some critics have argued that recognizing a right to die would eventually result in viewing killing as a beneficent act. Edmund Pellegrino rejects the right to die for this very reason.[28] Once killing is seen as beneficent, there would be no way to distinguish between medical and nonmedical interventions. The patient's right to die has, as its corollary, the duty of a doctor to accede to this request. It might even mean that a patient has a *duty* to die under certain conditions.[29]

A further consequence of beneficent killing would be the rampant abuse of medical authority, such that patients could not be protected against discrimination. We would start to evaluate the patient's quality of life to determine whether it would be better for her to live or die. This slippery slope could even result in the terrifying legitimation of *involuntary* euthanasia.

This concern is valid. Any evaluation of a patient's quality of life, especially if he is not terminally ill, would indeed put pressure on both patients and doctors. We are not good judges of whether suffering is unbearable, nor should we concern ourselves with determining who is fit to live. On my view, however, PAS prevents this slippery slope; it does not cause it. PAS could be a carefully circumscribed option for qualified patients rather than a general right to die. Under these conditions, it matters how the death is achieved: whether a patient competently self-administers the fatal dose or whether the doctor does it for them.

In the discussion of the doctrine of double effect, I argued that we tend to be preoccupied with the metaphysics of causing a death. In other words, a doctor does not cause a death in the context of CSD because the underlying disease is what kills the patient. But in the context of PAS, we should be similarly interested in whether the patient actively administers the dose or passively receives it. Pellegrino, like Velleman, is too comfortable conflating physician-assisted suicide with euthanasia.

If PAS is a unique action done by uniquely qualified patients, then it is implausible to believe that it would lead to viewing killing as beneficent. Nor would it lead to involuntary euthanasia because the patient requesting a fatal dose of barbiturates is *not* granting the doctor permission to perform the action. Unlike CSD, she is fully conscious and not yet experiencing the kind of intractable pain that would cloud her ability to consent.

These special qualifications and not a general judgment of the quality of life make PAS a morally legitimate option. So this carefully carved exception would not lead to a more expansive right and the discrimination that could inevitably follow. Making assisted death a general right would involve another false equivalence between the standpoint of the terminally ill, imminently dying patient and someone who fits neither of those criteria. Once again, we see substantial evidence of our failure to appreciate a specific and narrowly defined end-of-life dilemma.

The concern about beneficent killing and involuntary euthanasia is an important lesson for right-to-die advocates. They risk undermining their own goals when they advocate for "death with dignity." This is exactly the kind of vague description that could make killing seem benevolent and involuntary euthanasia legitimate. Opponents of suicide, like Immanuel Kant, have used this exact term to suggest that killing oneself is the ultimate undignified act.

The assumption here is that a life can be meaningless and should be allowed to end in a dignified fashion. My view, by way of contrast, is that we cannot meaningfully call the CSD alternative a life at all. It does not matter whether one subscribes to the higher-brain definition of death or just recognizes that CSD is its functional equivalent for the patient. This is *not* a claim about a patient's quality of life but rather an insistence that the patient, as a person, is no longer alive. So it has no implications for judging anyone else's quality of life. It does not put society on the slippery slope to discrimination, beneficent killing, and even involuntary euthanasia.

A carefully carved PAS exception is not a simple exercise in control. Rather, it is in response to the massive amount of control that doctors and proxies *already* have in end-of-life dilemmas. The psychology behind such a request is plausibly described, at least for some patients, as one of Stoic acceptance. This acceptance is not an attitude of sad resignation. It is something that opponents of physician-assisted suicide do not seem capable of comprehending. In fact, the New York Task Force issued the following recommendation for doctors dealing with a PAS request: "When a patient requests assisted suicide or euthanasia, a health care professional should explore the significance of the request, recognize the patient's suffering, and seek to discover the factors leading to the request. These factors may include insufficient symptom control, clinical depression, inadequate social support, concern about burdening family or others, hopelessness, loss of self-esteem, or fear of abandonment."[30]

One consideration is conspicuously absent from this long list of possible concerns: the confrontation with one's own mortality. Try as we might to reduce this existential dilemma to the symptoms by which it is manifested, we fail to grasp the patient's perspective. We should readily admit this and honestly explore its implications. Instead, we exert profound control over end-of-life dilemmas. We force the patient into the position of the dog being dragged by the moving wagon instead of allowing her to find some peace in accepting her fate.

NOTES

1. In lieu of visiting the New Orleans Pharmacy Museum, you can read about this story and others at http://www.pharmacymuseum.org/about, accessed April 21, 2016. I do not know why there was a twelve-year gap between the establishment of a licensing exam and Dufilho's landmark achievement. Next time I go on the tour, I will ask.
2. Johann Hari writes extensively about the Harrison Act in *Chasing the Scream: The First and Last Days of the War on Drugs* (New York: Bloomsburg, 2015).
3. For an excellent synopsis and analysis of this case, see Ian McColl Kennedy, "The Karen Quinlan Case: Problems and Proposals," *Journal of Medical Ethics* 2 (1976): 3-7.
4. Some fascinating correspondence from doctors and lawyers about this case can be found in "Correspondence," the *New England Journal of Medicine* 324 (1991): 561-62.
5. For an interesting analysis of the *Cruzan* case, see Michael Rie, "Practicing Medicine, Fiduciary Trust Privacy, and Public Moral Interloping after '*Cruzan*,'" *Journal of Medicine and Philosophy* 17, no. 6 (1992): 647-64.
6. Jim Salter, "Missouri Governor Halts First U.S. Execution by Propofol," *Washington Post*, October 11, 2013, accessed November 7, 2015, https://www.washingtonpost.com/politics/missouri-gov-halts-1st-us-execution-by-propofol/2013/10/11/559e6af6-32d9-11e3-8627-c5d7de0a046b_story.html.
7. Fred Barbash, "After 18 Botched IV Attempts on a Screaming, Bleeding Inmate, Ohio Gets Another Chance to Execute Him," *Washington Post*, March 17, 2016, accessed August 1, 2016, https://www.washingtonpost.com/news/morning-mix/wp/2016/03/17/after-18-botched-iv-attempts-on-a-screaming-bleeding-inmate-ohio-gets-another-chance-to-execute-him/.
8. Barbash, "After 18 Botched IV Attempts," 2016.
9. Astrid Galvan and Justin Pritchard, "Feds Confiscate Lethal-Injection Drugs Obtained Overseas by Arizona and Texas," *U.S. News and World Report*, October 23, 2015, accessed March 4, 2015, http://www.usnews.com/news/us/articles/2015/10/23/documents-arizona-tried-to-illegally-import-execution-drug.
10. See American Medical Association, "Ethical Opinion E-2.06: Capital Punishment," *Code of Medical Ethics of the American Medical Association* (Chicago: American Medical Association, 2006), 19-20.
11. Wayne Sumner, "And When I Die: The Pro-Life Case for Assisted Suicide," October 15, 2014, accessed December 3, 2014, http://thewalrus.ca/and-when-i-die/.
12. Michael O. Hardimon, *Hegel's Social Philosophy: The Project of Reconciliation* (Cambridge: Cambridge University Press, 1994), 85.
13. Gregory Hays, Introduction to Marcus Aurelius, *Meditations*, trans. Gregory Hays (New York: Modern Library, 2003), xx-xxi.
14. For instance, Epictetus councils his reader to think of his dead child as a broken cup. See Epictetus, *The Enchiridion, or Handbook* (Auckland: Floating Press, 2009): xxvi.
15. I have much more to say about the conflation of "personal" with "merely subjective" in my discussion of pedagogy in chapter 6.
16. J. David Velleman, "Against the Right to Die," *Journal of Medicine and Philosophy* 17 (1992): 665.

17. Velleman, "Against the Right to Die," 671-72.
18. Velleman, "Against the Right to Die," 673.
19. Velleman, "Against the Right to Die," 675.
20. I explain this concept in the sentences that follow this reference. But for additional reading, see Barry Schwartz, *The Paradox of Choice: Why Less Is More, rev. ed.* (New York: HarperCollins, 2016).
21. Velleman, "Against the Right to Die," 673.
22. Rachelle E. Bernacki and Susan D. Block, "Communication about Serious Illness Care Goals: A Review and Synthesis of Best Practices," *JAMA Internal Medicine* 174, no.12 (December 2014): 1998.
23. A study conducted by the Stanford University School of Medicine supports this line of argument from the perspective of doctors. See Tracie White, "Most Physicians Would Forgo Aggressive Treatment for Themselves at the End of Life, Study Finds," *Stanford Medicine News Center*, May 28, 2014, accessed July 16, 2016, https://med.stanford.edu/news/all-news/2014/05/most-physicians-would-forgo-aggressive-treatment-for-themselves-.html.
24. Richard M. Doerflinger and Carlos Gomez, "Killing the Pain Not the Patient: Palliative Care vs. Assisted Suicide," *United States Conference of Catholic Bishops*, accessed March 10, 2016, http://www.usccb.org/about/pro-life-activities/respect-life-program/killing-the-pain.cfm.
25. New York Task Force on Life and the Law, "When Death Is Sought—Assisted Suicide and Euthanasia in the Medical Context," Executive Summary, 1994, accessed January 4, 2015, https://www.health.ny.gov/regulations/task_force/reports_publications/when_death_is_sought/preface.htm.
26. New York Task Force, "When Death Is Sought."
27. New York Task Force, "When Death Is Sought."
28. See especially Edmund Pellegrino, "The False Promise of Beneficent Killing," in *Regulating How We Die: The Ethical, Medical, and Legal Issues Surrounding Physician-Assisted Suicide*, ed. Linda Emanuel (Cambridge, MA: Harvard University Press, 1998), 71-91.
29. See John Hardwig, ed., *Is There a Duty to Die? And Other Essays in Bioethics* (New York: Routledge, 2000).
30. New York Task Force, "When Death is Sought."

Part III

Chapter Five

Bones, Sinews, and the Self

The *Phaedo* is an ancient dialogue concerning the nature of the soul and the prospects for its immortality. Plato's account takes place after Socrates's conviction, and it culminates with him self-administering the fatal dose of hemlock. In an important but underappreciated digression, Socrates discusses the nature of causality. He refers to the philosophy of Anaxagoras, whom he has heard attributes causal power to mind or *nous*. Upon reading Anaxagoras's account, however, he finds himself disappointed that the theory puts more weight on material explanations. Socrates then references his own circumstances in jail and awaiting death by way of analogy:

> That seemed to me much like saying that Socrates' actions are all due to his mind, and then in trying to tell the causes of everything I do, to say that the reason that I am sitting here is because my body consists of *bones and sinews*, because the bones are hard and are separated by joints, that the sinews are such as to contract and relax, that they surround the bones along with flesh and skin which hold them together, then as the bones are hanging in their sockets, the relaxation and contraction of the sinews enable me to bend my limbs, and that is the cause of my sitting here with my limbs bent. [1]

Socrates rejects a material explanation for his current condition. He is in jail because (rightly or wrongly) a jury of his peers convicted him of refusing to recognize the gods of the city and for corrupting the youth. A second and equally important reason is that Socrates refused to escape when Crito, his wealthy and influential friend, tried to persuade him to do so. These are rational explanations, and they have an explanatory power unmatched by any material description.

In the last chapter, I reframed debates over acceptance and control. I insisted that physician-assisted suicide redistributes the control that already exists for doctors and proxies and that it does so in a morally appropriate way. A carefully carved exception for PAS will not lead to discrimination, abuse, and even involuntary euthanasia. On the contrary, it is more likely to prevent these problems: Self-administering the fatal dose ensures that the patient is not a merely passive recipient of whatever doctors and proxies deem to be appropriate. Then I suggested that a terminally ill patient contemplating PAS might be described as having an attitude of Stoic acceptance rather than a desire to illicitly control her fate.

In this chapter, my task is to show how the distinction between persons and organisms is both morally crucial and under attack in profound ways. As I have argued, patient values have already been undermined by the compelled consent to continuous sedation until death. We do not take a patient's conscious consent seriously enough, even though that particular patient is the one forced to face her own mortality. But beyond this problem of informed consent, I am concerned that consciousness *itself* is at risk of eventually being declared by neuroscience to be an illusion. So in this chapter, I offer my own slippery-slope argument about the unmasking of consciousness and the ultimate erosion of patient consent.

My alternative to this reductive physiological approach is a practical conception of consciousness that survives any attempt to reduce it to its physical properties. The first-person standpoint is ineradicable *for me*, even if scientific advances could ultimately undermine consciousness, personhood, and consent in general. Whether we care about this first-person perspective or not is an ethical decision, not a scientific conclusion.

This view is consistent with recognizing the need for a PAS option: Permitting PAS establishes a firewall to prevent the undermining of a patient's consciousness at the end of life. It refutes the notion that continuous sedation until death could ever be an adequate option on its own. In fact, making CSD an inevitable outcome rather than a genuine choice sets the stage for an attack on consciousness and consent in end-of-life dilemmas. It fails to countenance the possibility that inducing a permanent loss of consciousness is a morally meaningful action.

In these exceptional cases, we should not shift moral significance onto an organism. Or we are at least owed an argument for the sanctity of the brain stem. Nor should we permit doctors and proxies to have unfettered control after a patient refuses treatment. We claim to care about the patient as a self-conscious *person* at every point until the patient refuses treatment. We are legally and morally obligated to do so based on the need to obtain informed consent. The manner and timing of death should be no different.

In the *Phaedo*, Socrates functions as Plato's metaphysical mouthpiece, and the relevant alternative to bones and sinews is a transcendent soul. One is free to accept or reject the logic of Socrates's (or perhaps Plato's) arguments for immortality. We can substitute consciousness for soul, and the insight remains the same. As we saw in chapter 2, consciousness could be adequately described as an emergent property, a special function that results from a physiological process. In other words, minds emerge from brains, but the special function that results might not be explicable in purely physiological terms. In this way, the rejection of a "bones and sinews" attitude toward consciousness does not commit one to any spiritual or supernatural claims. In fact, as I also argued in chapter 2, the higher-brain model of death (i.e., the irreversible loss of consciousness) offers a competing view of what makes an organism *what it is*. In this way, it functions on the same level as any physiological approach to these questions.

At the heart of Socrates's complaint about the way in which Anaxagoras confused rational and material explanations is the idea that human beings value rational intelligibility. For instance, when we ask *why* someone is sad, the claim that one's serotonin levels are askew is not an adequate response. Set aside the clear misrepresentation of brain chemistry. After all, the brain is not like a car that is low on fluids and needs to be topped off by a mechanic. A purely physiological explanation might account for the efficacy of a psychiatric drug, but it could never answer the kinds of questions that we, as persons, ask one another. We seek reasons for beliefs and actions (e.g., I am sad because my dog died this morning) and not simply biological reports on the status of one's brain chemistry. In this specific context, material explanations cannot do the work of rational accounts.

But what if this rational account is really just a myth? It could simply be the articulation of a folk-psychological belief that has no real referent in the external world.[2] Folk psychology is a commonsense, jargon-less way of attributing mental states to myself and to others. For instance, we might say that Sally intentionally punched Bob in the arm because she was offended by his joke. In the course of ordinary experience, this attribution is easily understood. It could even count as a rational explanation: If the punch was truly intentional and not an accident, then there must have been some motive or *reason* for Sally's behavior.

Various philosophers articulate some materialist position on this question. Perhaps the most reductive of these views is eliminative materialism. It claims that folk psychology provides us with a remedial and unscientific way of making sense of human behavior. The real explanation for my behavior pertains to my C fibers firing and not to my own claim about why I yelped in pain when I stubbed my toe. Even to call them "my" C fibers is to misleadingly make personal the effects of a complicated and impersonal physiological process. On this view, developments in neuroscience can (and will) help us to overcome these naïve assertions about human behavior.

Suppose that neuroscience could provide a purely physiological description of what happens when someone becomes an enraged highway driver. If rational explanations are really just folk-psychological descriptions, then the motives and intentions we attribute to this person are useful fictions. If the road rage leads to violence, then we call it malicious behavior. But malice does not describe any physiological process, so it does not have an actual referent. It might describe the feelings that we have about what happened, but introspection does not produce verifiable truth. On the other hand, knowing the physiological mechanisms that produce certain emotions could allow us to reliably predict (and even control) their manifestation.

One noteworthy consequence of this approach to consciousness is that it might undermine the doctrine of double effect. As we have seen, the DDE relies upon a meaningful distinction between foreseeing and intending. But if attributions of intent are folk-psychological fictions, then they cannot play a major role in an ethical theory. If the DDE is invalidated by advances in modern science, then there would be no meaningful difference between physician-assisted suicide and continuous sedation until death. The intent behind the action would be a fiction added to what was actually done. So the way in which end-of-life dilemmas are framed would look quite different.

Also, there might not even *be* a coherent definition of suicide as distinct from any other form of killing. The examples of CTE and PTSD that I discussed in chapter 3 could be used to show that the cause of suicide is a malfunctioning organism, a broken brain. Dave Duerson's "decision" to shoot himself in the chest, thereby preserving his brain for science, might attest to the fact that he was *compelled* to end his life in this way. The fact that it was done deliberately and with foresight is not enough to show that he was freely motivated to do so. And even if we find or attribute a motive, it would be but a superficial gloss on a purely physiological process.

The insights of contemporary neuroscience build on a long-running debate in the history of philosophy over the ontological status of consciousness and its relationship to personal identity. Some versions of a materialist response to this problem are ancient, as are their implications. On these views, it becomes difficult or even meaningless to talk about a *self* independent of its many manifestations. If there is no ghost in the machine, then perhaps all we are left with are the inner workings and outward effects of the machine itself.

Perhaps the self could still be, as David Hume puts it, a bundle of impressions, even if it is not a substance of its own.[3] It is no wonder that eliminative materialists like Patricia Churchland invoke Hume when they discuss the ethical implications of their research.[4] But it is reasonable to ask whether a bundle theory of the self could support a robust theory of individual autonomy. If a self is just a bundle of impressions, then why should it enjoy any ontological or epistemic priority?

As eliminative materialists are working to dispel folk-psychological views about the *contents* of consciousness, other philosophers argue that consciousness *itself* is an illusion. The so-called easy problem of consciousness can be solved by locating a neural mechanism for any particular function of the brain. As our ability to map the brain improves, this will not pose any special challenge. However, the "hard problem" of consciousness requires explaining how and why we experience ourselves as *self*-conscious beings. Why didn't human beings evolve to behave identically as we do right now but without any inner self-awareness or the feeling that we have freely chosen to behave in this way?[5]

One possible response is to claim that consciousness itself is just a trick of the brain. On this view, the contents of our introspection are folk-psychological fictions, but so is the idea of introspection itself. We *feel* as though we experience the world in a self-conscious way, but perhaps scientific advances could dispel this notion. Why should we assume that self-consciousness lies outside the purview of science, when any other phenomenon can be analyzed and understood? Appealing to the mysterious nature of introspection, then, would be nothing but an enormous argument from ignorance: Something must be the way we believe it to be simply because it has not yet been fully explained. The legal and moral implications of this proposed solution to the hard problem of consciousness go far beyond undermining agent intention: There is no agent even to intend the action but only complex neural activity. We would still reward or punish the activity, but we would be factually incorrect to attribute it to a person who freely and deliberately willed it.

If this all sounds too futuristic and speculative, here is a present-day example of how such a system of punishment might function. Darren Sharper was a Super Bowl champion safety for the New Orleans Saints. After his retirement, he parlayed his celebrity into an active social life. Only later did it surface that Sharper used this as an opportunity to drug, sexually assault, and rape nine women in four different states. After his eventual release from prison, the revised plea deal stipulates that Sharper must undergo "penile plethysmograph" exams, while on lifetime probation.[6] This instrument is designed to gauge sexual arousal: A sensor is attached to the penis, and a series of sexual images flashes by. A machine designed to measure his physiological response to stimuli will determine whether Mr. Sharper is ever deemed to be rehabilitated. At no point will his self-conscious testimony truly matter. Nor will, we might presume, the attestations of medical experts (at least when they contradict the data). A carefully calibrated machine can provide us with the answer.

These exams might remind you of an infamous scene in *A Clockwork Orange*, were it not for the fact that Mr. Sharper will (presumably) have free and unclamped use of his eyes.[7] If such a contraption truly works, then perhaps it makes sense to use it to determine whether someone is an unreformed and still-violent sexual predator. But we should do so with a full understanding of this new legal and moral terrain. It is not only the efficacy of physiological reports that we should be worried about; it is also what their use might mean for the idea of personhood.

***

In the last chapter, I discussed the concern that physician-assisted suicide will lead to discrimination, abuse, and even involuntary euthanasia. My response was twofold: First, these concerns apply to the claim that PAS should be a right but not to the idea that we could carefully carve a PAS exception for specific patients. A general right to die could (and likely would) be expanded indefinitely. But this is not true for a strictly delineated exception. Second, the passive nature of continuous sedation until death makes it prone to the same kind of abuse that a right to die might elicit. As we saw, even in the famous cases that established a right to refuse treatment, proxies and doctors *already* had control over the situation. So this crucial individual right was ironically established only *after* the respective patients were already permanently unconscious. In the case of CSD, as I have argued, it is dishonest and even dangerous to refuse to acknowledge that something more than a loss of social interaction or "subjective death" is occurring. This is especially worrisome when the actions undertaken on behalf of the patient are presumed to be beneficent.

If we take the conscious consent of a patient seriously, *as we are required to do by the need for informed consent*, then we cannot avoid asking hard questions about end-of-life dilemmas. However, we seem incapable of overcoming our "bones and sinews" approach to these dilemmas. As we have already seen, the whole-brain or cardiopulmonary definitions of death in fact introduce new philosophical problems that do not surface in the same way if a patient opts for PAS. If a patient avails herself of a PAS option, then the person (minimally defined as the capacity for consciousness) and the organism die simultaneously. So there is no one left to be benefitted or harmed by future medical interventions. As the ancient philosopher Epicurus noted, "Why should I fear death? If I am, then death is not. If death is, then I am not."[8] The basic idea is that the dead cannot be harmed because there is no longer a subject to be harmed.

But what should we say about the prospect of harming someone (if we can even use the word *someone*) who has been continuously sedated until death? Even if you reject the higher-brain criterion for death, it is clear that *something* has happened to the patient. If we refuse to call it death, then we would still have to admit that the self or subject or person is not to be found. If the dead cannot be harmed because there is no subject to be harmed, then what is the difference between an action done to someone who has undergone an irreversible loss of consciousness and someone whose organism is also dead? In either case, no subject is there to be harmed.

We might even call this a strange case of "wrongful life." When a child is born with a serious impairment that went undiagnosed in the womb, some believe that the child should eventually be permitted to sue the medical testing company or even her own parents.[9] The claim is not that the impairment could have been remedied but rather that the child would have been better off not existing at all. So the parents or the testing company are being accused of negligently forcing existence on the person.

In the case of end-of-life dilemmas, the argument might take a similar form. The whole-brain defense of CSD creates a scenario under which the organism is compelled to outlive the person. Aside from the question of what moral status this "unconscious life" has, the patient believes that it is better for the organism to die with the person. This type of forced existence would, on her view, count as wrongful life. In other words, she would concede that her personhood would have already been terminated, but she would object to the continued existence of her organism.

A terminally ill patient thinking prospectively about CSD might have good reason to fear the wrongful imposition of this morally ambiguous form of life. Her loved ones would not be wrong to agonize over her unconscious organism, *having already witnessed the withering away of her consciousness*. To them, it is still *her* in a way. So her fear is reasonable because she realizes that the reaction of her loved ones is rational in its own way.

This dilemma is not unique to cases of CSD. The infamous Terry Schiavo controversy illustrates the legal and moral melee that can occur whenever a organism outlives a person.[10] The fact that Terry's organism was animated does not make her case categorically different from a case of continuous sedation until death. Nor does it matter how much time it takes for the organism to perish in either case. Both examples deal with the question of how to regard a permanently unconscious organism. Regrettably, the Schiavo example also shows the shameful moral and political jockeying that can accompany such a scenario.

The fact that CSD uniquely creates new and strange dilemmas runs counter to what its defenders preach. James Bernat, for instance, insists that the higher-brain model muddles up our tidy, empirically grounded definitions. It does this by introducing vague and empirically unverifiable concepts like personhood. On his view, "a higher vertebrate organism can reside in only one of two states, alive or dead: no organism can be in both states or in neither."[11]

This observation is almost tautologous in its reasoning. For this very reason, it tells us virtually nothing about death. The higher-brain view does not entail an organism being both dead and alive at the same time. Rather, it suggests that the person and the organism are ontologically distinct entities. A person is dead when there is a permanent and irreversible loss of consciousness. The organism, however, can survive this death. As I argued earlier, this can create moral uncertainty for the patient and her family. This confusion is underwritten by the whole-brain approach, which stipulates that the patient is still alive, only unconscious.

The higher-brain model involves no such uncertainty, as it sharply distinguishes between the deaths of two different ontological entities: the person and the organism. The organism and the person can be practically related while also being ontologically distinct. For example, the brain is required for consciousness. Also, as we have seen, the highest degree of emergent function might ultimately depend upon the presence of consciousness. The research I referenced in chapter 2 suggests that the brain activity of a fully conscious patient with locked-in syndrome is qualitatively different from the brain activity of a patient who is comatose. Any claim about the status of an *organism* will involve some degree of judgment. And, again, a patient can be declared dead by the whole-brain model before their organs have failed. Having functioning organs, then, is a necessary but not sufficient condition to be a human organism. Those who advocate for the higher-brain model simply go one step further: Some *specific* brain functions are required for an organism to be fully integrated. This does not include the brain stem.

If this nascent view is corroborated by developments in neuroscience, then it would be question begging to attempt to define death for all "higher vertebrate organisms." We would need to know more about the degree to which an organism has the capacity for consciousness. None of this investigation would be mere conjecture; it would be grounded in an analysis of the brain.

Let us grant for the sake of argument that the whole-brain model is the least risky definition of death. Given our current technology and knowledge of the brain, it is true that diagnosing an irreversible loss of consciousness might lead to false positives in declaring a patient dead. This is the most compelling reason to opt for a view that relies upon a flatlining EEG. However, *even if* the whole-brain option were the best, this would not show that CSD is its required outcome. There is no risk of a false positive when a patient self-administers the fatal dose. Having a PAS option could be recognized as a reasonable and necessary *exception* to the typical way in which we view persons and organisms. But so long as we maintain our preoccupation with the status of the brain stem, we cannot recognize a meaningful alternative to our current "bones and sinews" approach to death.

***

Eliminative materialists, along with those who believe that we can explain the hard problem of consciousness, make bold claims about the scope of scientific explanation. But perhaps the only reason these claims seem bold is because this area of scientific inquiry is still in its infancy. So here is my version of a slippery-slope argument: Suppose that we continue to map the brain in the same way that we have decoded the human genome. We pile up the evidence for solving the easy problem of consciousness, and then we make a breakthrough into understanding the hard problem. This assumes that self-consciousness is, in principle, explainable (and I wonder if this is actually the case). Still, neuroscientists will present various solutions to the problem, and some of them might be compelling.

This modern version of causation by "bones and sinews" would pose a huge problem for the ethical requirement that we obtain informed consent. If intentions, and even agents themselves, are illusions that can be explained away, then why should we concern ourselves with them? Although the DDE has a number of flaws, especially when applied to end-of-life dilemmas, at least it puts *some* check on what persons in power can do to passive bodies. If informed consent can be called into question in general, scientific advances might pose a special problem for patients whose decision would cause their death. It is not difficult to imagine that we could prize the efficacy of treatment over patient goals, even though this is an ethical and not an empirical question.

Let us reconsider an example that I have used several times before: the right of a Jehovah's Witness to refuse a blood transfusion, even if it results in his death. Parents cannot refuse a blood transfusion for their children, so this right applies only to an individual who holds the relevant belief. We deem it to be an invasion of one's conscience, a violation of one's sincerely held beliefs, to force this treatment upon an individual. But why should we respect this form of introspection and personal testimony once science shows that it is so much hot air? We already have some methods for determining whether someone is being sincere, and we will continue to refine them.[12] It is not wildly speculative to suggest that the belief itself could be physiologically undermined. If an organism needs new blood in order to survive, then the medical experts who can facilitate this might eventually be permitted to do so. Doctors, as mechanics of the body, will attend to the health of the organism. There is no person inhabiting the organism, or at least no person whose subjective and illusory preferences should trump medical expertise.

This example is important because it combines 1) the assumption that persons should want to live; 2) the fact that blood transfusions easily and painlessly satisfy this outcome; and 3) the need, in spite of that, to respect sincerely held religious beliefs. There is no doubt that religious belief is an especially protected form of conscious assent in the United States. Yet one wonders how it would fare against advances in neuroscience. Religious freedom might not be so sacrosanct and inviolable once we discover the neurological mechanisms that produce religious belief.[13] This is especially relevant for beliefs (like the prohibition on donating, storing, and transfusing blood) that are *already* regarded by the majority as counterintuitive or even irrational. Perhaps one reason the right to refuse a blood transfusion does not extend to one's children is because we do not want to socially sanction such an eccentric belief. If we could scientifically undermine and even eliminate this belief entirely, many of us would be tempted to do so.

The way in which we have framed end-of-life dilemmas makes us especially vulnerable to the kinds of scientific advances that could undermine the need to procure informed consent. We have defined both death and medicine in purely physiological terms, excluding by fiat the role that consciousness might legitimately play in both accounts. Death cannot involve a permanent loss of consciousness, even though this is at least functionally equivalent to death for the patient herself. Continuous sedation counts as medicine, even though it achieves its goals of symptom relief by eradicating the consciousness that could experience pain. In both cases, there is a general disregard for the way in which a patient consciously approaches her own mortality.

One way of escaping this dilemma is to deny that mental states could be reduced to their physical properties. So the thoughts, beliefs, and intentions of conscious persons could not be fully accounted for scientifically. This would give us a way of prioritizing the patient's perspective, even in the midst of massive advances in neuroscience. Philosophers of mind and cognitive scientists have designed various thought experiments to press this point. Perhaps the most famous of these experiments is the one proposed by Frank Jackson. In a series of articles in the 1980s, Jackson presents the case of Mary, a scientist who knows all of the physiological properties and neural mechanisms associated with the perception of color.[14] However, she is confined to a black-and-white room, and she conducts her investigations solely with the use of a black-and-white television monitor.

Jackson asks whether a scientist with Mary's amount of knowledge would *learn* anything about color if she were to leave the room or be given a monitor that broadcasts the world beyond black and white. He concludes that Mary surely would learn something new. For the first time, she would learn what it is like to have a subjective experience of color. But if this is so, then we must recognize the existence of nonphysical attributes that might be called qualia. We must also concede that we cannot have a completely physical or material explanation for conscious experience.

There have been many different lines of argument for and against Jackson's conclusion. The relevant point here is that this thought experiment gives us a way to establish the existence of nonphysical properties that cannot be analyzed scientifically. So even if we discover the neural mechanisms underlying, for example, a sincerely held religious belief, we could never know scientifically what it is like to subjectively hold such a belief. There is something ineffable about human experience that reveals the limits of scientific investigation.

However, I wonder if a defense of *qualia* could ever survive the kinds of scientific advances that we have assumed for the sake of discussion. We have already granted that neuroscience is still in its infancy, so why are we entitled to assume that it could never account for subjective experience? As in the earlier discussion of introspection, I am not sure how we can avoid making another enormous argument from ignorance. It might be true right now that we cannot understand qualia, but that does not mean that we never could. Similarly, it seems to beg the question to stipulate that Mary "knows everything there is to know" scientifically about color but that she is missing the subjective experience. This seems to rule out the very *possibility* of scientifically accounting for subjective experience, when this was supposed to be the conclusion of the argument.[15]

Discussing the subjective element of experience in terms of nonphysical properties makes this idea seem almost pseudoscientific. It reifies a personal experience, invents a new term for it, makes it seem like the kind of thing that could be understood, and then insists that science cannot do so. Since science is in the business of analyzing phenomena, this seems like a wrong-headed strategy. It is also, I think, unnecessary and beside the point. We could grant the supposition that neuroscience will eventually give us a complete scientific account of human experience. But we could then defend consciousness as a practical standpoint, a way in which experiences become meaningful and valuable *for a particular person*. This would hold regardless of whether science could ultimately explain qualia.

For example, even if it were true that the content of one's sincerely held religious beliefs could be completely understood neurologically, we could still respect the fact that those beliefs are meaningful and valuable *for that particular person*. Suppose that neuroscience progresses so much that we completely dispel the concept of *qualia* and even solve the hard problem of consciousness. Suppose further that we study the brain of a monk using sophisticated imaging that is far more advanced than current fMRI technology. None of these scientific breakthroughs help us to *ethically* evaluate the monk's insistence that his religious beliefs are personal and sacred.

Perhaps Mary would not, in fact, learn anything new by leaving the black-and-white room or by having her monitor upgraded. Color would have a different significance for her, but she would gain no new propositional knowledge about it. Whether we care about how meaningful her beliefs are *for her* or not is an ethical and not a scientific judgment.

Now suppose that Mary is a world-famous oncologist. She knows everything there is to know scientifically about the effects of cancer on the body, but with one important exception: She does not know how to cure it. Mary starts to develop what she immediately recognizes as the symptoms of an aggressive and ultimately terminal form of cancer. Her scientific expertise allows her to diagnose these symptoms, as well as to determine her prognosis. It does not, however, offer *any* guidance for how to interpret this evidence *in light of her own values*. No truth claims could even be made about how she ultimately decides to respond to this news. We could care to value the meaning of the diagnosis for the patient, or we could not care. Either way, there would be no implications whatsoever for our scientific understanding or for claims about what is true and real.

There is nothing factually incoherent about dispelling Mary's intentions as mere illusions. Nor is it somehow inconsistent to view Mary herself as a complicated series of neural connections. Still, these judgments could both be *unethical*. The scientific explanation could be perfect, but it would still not tell us how to evaluate the meaning and value of Mary's subjective experience. This is true even if the experience itself can be fully explained, all the way down to the qualia. In other words, once the scientific debate over the truth value of subjective experience plays out, we are still left with the ethical question of whether to care about the meaning and value of the experience *for the patient*.

We could take the argument one step further. There is nothing in science that prevents us from regarding one another as mere automata (to use Descartes's famous image).[16] And it might prove to be *more* scientifically consistent to treat one another as zombies who outwardly resemble conscious beings in every way but who utterly lack self-consciousness.[17] This would be true on the assumption that eliminative materialism proves to be correct and that the hard problem of consciousness is ultimately explained. But none of this even begins to address the ethical question of how to regard the meaning and value of subjective experience once it has been scientifically explained.

This observation is not an attempt to dodge a difficult scientific question. Rather, it is a way of dissolving, or at least circumscribing, its ethical significance. Recall for a moment the example of Stoic freedom from the last chapter: Even if one's fate has absolutely already been determined, interpreting the meaning and value of this fact is completely up to oneself. Now imagine that *even* this interpretation could be explained scientifically. It is not hard to imagine. Perhaps a patient with a pessimistic temperament has a brain that fires in a certain way, whereas the inner workings of a different brain manifest in an optimistic outlook. Set aside the question of whether one can voluntarily change the way in which one's brain functions. The source of one's temperament has no *practical* significance for a patient who finds herself to be pessimistic or hopeful. She finds herself with that temperament regardless, and whether we respect her attitude and outlook is not at all a scientific question.

One response to this claim might take the following form: If 1) scientific analysis can prove or disprove the reality of mental contents (like intention) and even of consciousness itself, and if 2) truth claims are also meaningful, then 3) the results of scientific inquiry must have a practical impact. In other words, one cannot hypothetically grant to science as much as I already have but then insist that questions of meaning and value are not affected by its conclusions. So it would matter whether the terminally ill patient's preferences originate from a *self* or whether they result from a physiological process. We would have no reason to honor a patient's preference were it to be nothing more than the manifestation of a complex physiological process.

In response to this concern, I would suggest that this line of argument conflates scientific and ethical questions. We have good *ethical* reasons for not treating each other as automata or as unconscious zombies, *regardless* of what science ultimately proves. Even in cases of severe mental illness, where a person's behavior can be explained by a malfunction of the brain, we still owe the patient a high degree of moral regard. We ought not to think of her solely as a malfunctioning brain, even if we could perfectly predict and control her responses to stimuli. Having scientific sanction to treat others as mere automata or as unconscious zombies does not make this dehumanizing treatment morally correct.

Further, our ability to treat other persons in this way does not extend to our own *self*-regard. Adopting this attitude toward others might be scientifically plausible or even preferable, but it is morally repugnant. When it comes to our own self-understanding, we cannot coherently view ourselves as complex machines in the same way. We might imaginatively adopt a third-person perspective on our given situation, just as Mary the oncologist can diagnose her own symptoms. But when it comes to questions of meaning and value, we cannot entirely escape the first-person perspective. These values are *mine*, whether they have chemical origins or not. This is especially true when my own mortality is at issue.

***

It is true that we can, over time and with great effort, mitigate what David Foster Wallace called our "natural, hard-wired default setting, which is to be deeply and literally self-centered, and to see and interpret everything through this lens of self."[18] Here he is making an epistemological rather than an ethical claim. At issue is not whether human beings are naturally selfish in a moral sense but rather the fact that each individual occupies but one perspective, a single standpoint, instead of having a view of the whole: "There is no experience you've had that you were not at the absolute center of. The world as you experience it is right there in front of you, or behind you, to the left or right of you, on your TV, or your monitor, or whatever. Other people's thoughts and feelings have to be communicated to you somehow, but your own are so immediate, urgent, *real*."[19]

This epistemological point precedes any ethical evaluation. We could choose to care or not to care about the thoughts and feelings that others must communicate to us. However, we do not make a choice *in the same way* about our own thoughts and feelings. Foster Wallace made these comments in the context of a commencement speech titled "This Is Water." The speech begins with the following story: "There are these two young fish swimming along, and they happen to meet an older fish swimming the other way, who nods at them and says, ‘Morning, boys, how’s the water?’ And the two young fish swim on for a bit, and then eventually one of them looks over at the other and goes, ‘What the hell is water?’”[20]

As we mature and become more reflective, we learn that each singular perspective is but a pinpoint in a much larger context. So the lens of self through which I interpret the world is one perspective on an infinitely bigger picture. But recognizing this does not make deeply held views and values *false* for the person holding them. For instance, the fact that a devout Hindu was born and raised in a culture that supports or even produces such a belief does not invalidate that person’s religious commitment. Assuming that we could explain away an individual’s deeply held belief by identifying its underlying cause is to commit a basic genetic fallacy. The meaning of a belief for any particular person is distinct from the source that may or may not have produced it. Likewise, the older fish can recognize that he is swimming in water. But this does not mean that he could survive outside of it.

Try as we might, we cannot fully adopt the insights of science into our own self-understanding. In order to do so, we would need to be able to view our own lives impersonally and from a third-person perspective. When we witness someone else stubbing his toe, we can explain his pain in terms of C fibers firing. When I stub my toe, I can say the same thing. But my experience of the pain remains, regardless of my scientific explanation. I might also attach meaning and value to it. Even the attempt to be as scientifically consistent and impartial as possible is motivated by the nonscientific judgment that it would be *better* for me to do so. So every time I stub my toe, I remind myself that my C fibers are firing. But this is just a way of striving to cultivate a new folk-psychological attitude rather than the total rejection of these attitudes as myths. And science cannot offer us any guidance for determining which folk-psychological attitudes are better and which are worse.

We cannot completely become the narrators of our own lives. In this way, we are condemned to subjectivity. An illustrative example of this is the attempt to contemplate the prospect of one’s own nonexistence. Sam Harris, the neuroscientist and public intellectual, invites us to undertake a thought experiment that purports to show just how easy it is to make our own mortality intelligible.[21] He asks us to imagine what it might be like in Paris, France, at this very moment. We can form a concept of a busy street, a baguette with butter and Brie, the Louvre. But none of this requires that we be in Paris presently. We might have never gone, nor may ever go, but life in Paris keeps on ticking whether we are there or not. By analogy, then, one’s own death obviously does not entail the end of the world. It is easy to imagine the world continuing without me, just as it had for the millennia before I was born.

Harris concludes that it is simply a lack of effort that prevents us from conceiving of our own nonexistence. However, I think that his conclusion is far-fetched and self-defeating. Forming a concept of Paris is easy, but imagining that I no longer exist is a real conceptual feat. It would suggest a remarkable, maybe even superhuman, capacity to regard our *own* lives as a narrator would a story. For example, imagining the permanent absence of a loved one is terribly painful but possible. We are still around to do the imagining, and our lives will continue, even if they are forever changed. Similarly, calling to mind a particular image of Paris (whether it is from one's own trip or from a magazine ad) is an ordinary act of consciousness. But it is something altogether different to engage in a thought experiment where the object of consciousness is its *own* complete and total absence. Harris's analogy might seem superficially plausible. But genuinely contemplating one's own mortality requires that we use the very capacity that we are imagining to be nonexistent.

One's perspective on one's own life and values is categorically distinct from the way in which one might scientifically and imaginatively regard other persons. However, the same ethical concerns apply to both cases. Whether we respect a patient's wishes, even after science has revealed them to be elaborate illusions, is an ethical and not a scientific question. But the insights of these modern versions of *bones and sinews* (e.g., eliminative materialism and solving the hard problem of consciousness) surely make it more tempting to reduce persons to organisms. We are already prepared to do so, given our stipulated definitions for death and for medicine. This is because we have carelessly conflated scientific and ethical concerns.

We could still avoid the slippery slope that undercuts the meaning and even existence of informed consent. This would require an ethical counterpunch to scientific claims. However, as we saw in chapter 3, the main ethical principle operative in end-of-life dilemmas (the DDE) concedes rather than challenges these scientific presumptions. It sanctions the claim that killing involves the death of the organism and not the person. Further, the DDE is *itself* undermined by the same scientific advances that threaten patient consent. It would be tempting not to care about agent intention if intent is a myth and the agent herself is an illusion.[22]

On my view, the way out of this dilemma is to build an ethical firewall against the creeping threats to consciousness. Suppose that we grant the ability of scientists to discover the neurological mechanisms for emotions and beliefs that we believe to be freely chosen. We could further grant that the self is not a unique substance or some reified being with special powers. Still, the fact that a particular patient regards herself as holding beliefs and values *of her own* seems morally relevant. One such belief is the idea that an irreversible loss of consciousness is a sufficient cause of death. This is intentionally and directly caused by both physician-assisted suicide and continuous sedation until death. One such value is that it is better for the organism not to survive the death of one's consciousness. This is uniquely achieved by PAS.

From a scientific perspective, it might be false to ascribe these beliefs to a conscious person. Perhaps they emanate from a complex and totally impersonal neurological process. Nonetheless, it matters that this process took place in this particular organism, with this particular consciousness as an emergent property. My own values cannot be an illusion *for me*, and this is true for any particular patient's own self-regard. We could still demand a respect for *persons*, even in a world where scientific advances have shown them to be illusions. I do not think, however, that our current conceptual framework for end-of-life dilemmas permits us to do so.

NOTES

1. Plato, *Phaedo*, in *Plato: Complete Works*, ed. John M. Cooper (Indianapolis: Hackett, 1997), 98c–98d, emphasis added.

2. See especially Paul Churchland, "Eliminative Materialism and the Propositional Attitudes," *Journal of Philosophy* (1981): 67–90.

3. David Hume, "Of Personal Identity," in *A Treatise of Human Nature*, ed. P.H. Nidditch (Oxford: Clarendon Oxford, 1973), Book I, Part 4, Section 6.

4. See especially Patricia Churchland, *Braintrust: What Neuroscience Tells Us about Morality* (Princeton: Princeton University Press, 2011).

5. The literature on this topic is extensive. A good place to start is with David J. Chalmers, "Facing Up to the Problem of Consciousness," *Journal of Consciousness Studies* 2, no. 3 (1995): 200–19.

6. John Simerman and Ramon Antonio Vargas, "'Penile Plethysmograph' Test to Gauge Arousal Part of Darren Sharper's Strict Post-Prison Deal," *New Orleans Advocate*, April 14, 2015, accessed June 5, 2016, http://www.theadvocate.com/new_orleans/news/article_a0ccb184-5acd-5508-bfec-6982605b5fac.html.

7. This is an iconic scene in Stanley Kubrick's film adaptation, but the original book is also well worth a read: Anthony Burgess, *A Clockwork Orange* (New York: W. W. Norton, 1995).

8. Epicurus, "Letter to Menoeceus," accessed September 17, 2014, http://www.epicurus.net/en/menoeceus.html.

9. For a captivating discussion of wrongful birth and wrongful life, see Wendy Hensel "The Disabling Impact of Wrongful Birth and Wrongful Life Actions," *Harvard Civil Rights–Civil Liberties Law Review* 40 (2005): 141–95.

10. See Arthur Caplan, James McCartney, and Dominic Sisti, eds., *The Case of Terri Schiavo: Ethics at the End of Life* (New York: Prometheus Books), 2006.

11. James Bernat, "The Whole-Brain Concept of Death Remains Optimum Public Policy," *Journal of Law, Medicine, and Ethics* 34, no. 1 (2006): 37.

12. Henry T. Greely discusses the implications of neuroscience for criminal justice in "The Neuroscience Revolution, Ethics, and the Law," April 20, 2004, accessed October 8, 2015, https://www.scu.edu/ethics/focus-areas/bioethics/resources/the-neuroscience-revolution-ethics-and-the-law/.

13. See Robert McCauley, *Why Religion Is Natural and Science Is Not* (Oxford: Oxford University Press, 2013).

14. Like the hard problem of consciousness, there is a mountain of literature on this topic. An excellent volume to explore would be Peter Ludlow, Yujim Nagasawa, and Daniel Stoljar, eds., *There's Something about Mary: Essays on Phenomenal Consciousness and Frank Jackson's Knowledge Argument* (Cambridge: MIT University Press, 2004).

15. This is one of the ways in which Daniel Dennett responds to Jackson's argument. See Howard Robinson, "Dennett on the Knowledge Argument," *Analysis* 53, no. 3 (July 1993): 174–77.

16. René Descartes, *Meditations on First Philosophy*, in *Discourse on Method and Meditations on First Philosophy*, trans. Donald Cress (Indianapolis: Hackett, 1998), 68.
17. Chalmers, "Facing Up."
18. David Foster Wallace, "This Is Water," *Transcription of the 2005 Kenyon Commencement Address*, May 21, 2005, accessed September 3, 2014, http://web.ics.purdue.edu/~drkelly/DFWKenyonAddress2005.pdf.
19. Wallace, "This Is Water."
20. Wallace, "This Is Water."
21. The Paris analogy comes from a debate on the topic "Does God Exist?" See "Sam Harris Debate with Rabbi David Wolpe," April 24, 2012, accessed May 28, 2016, https://www.youtube.com/watch?v=bN9nlAnkCUY. Another useful Harris video is titled "The Self Is an Illusion," *Big Think*, September 16, 2014, accessed March 5, 2015, https://www.youtube.com/watch?v=fajfkO_X0l0. Here Harris argues for the irreducibly subjective nature of consciousness, even as he claims that the self is an illusion. He endorses meditation as a way of overcoming this illusion, even though it is unclear who or what is being counseled to meditate.
22. Sam Harris ironically defends a version of the doctrine of double effect in his discussion of the ethics of war. But it is unclear why we should valorize agent intention if intent is, neuroscientifically speaking, a folk-psychological fiction. See Sam Harris and Omer Aziz, Waking Up Podcast #32, March 12, 2016, accessed July 30, 2017, https://www.samharris.org/podcast/item/the-best-podcast-ever.

Chapter Six

Pedagogy and the Limits of Ethics

In his incisive essay "Men without Chests," C. S. Lewis describes an important pedagogical dilemma. Lewis harshly criticizes the work of two pseudonymous authors of an elementary school textbook. His complaint is that the authors have unintentionally conveyed some provocative philosophical lessons about the nature of values. In particular, Lewis is concerned that students will subconsciously absorb the idea that all judgments of value are really just expressions of one's own *feelings*. So judging a waterfall to be "sublime," as the poet Coleridge does, is not to say anything about the waterfall itself.[1] Rather, it is merely to report one's own subjective experience.

The problem for Lewis that the poet's observation was not simply an articulation of his personal opinion. If that were true, then we could not even begin to have a conversation about values. We might, for a brief moment, feel secure in our solipsistic way of experiencing the world. However, we still want others to recognize the rational validity of our claims. So we make observations about the world as it is, and others may call upon us to defend our views. Solipsism might be a perfectly intelligible problem in a philosophy course, but it is not a remedy to competing claims about value in the real world. Insofar as it affects public life, we must at least attempt to hash this out through conversation or debate. Of course, we could be wrong (or only partially right) about our judgments, but this means that they are the kinds of things that we could get wrong in the first place.

Lewis does not believe that any of this was done deliberately. The authors of the textbook were also victims of a culture that frowns upon bold and objective declarations of value. This is true even though we expect rational adults to articulate and defend their views. Further, we expect them to behave as if there were such objective standards. Lewis writes,

> And all the time—such is the tragi-comedy of our situation—we continue to clamour for those very qualities we are rendering impossible. You can hardly open a periodical without coming across the statement that what our civilization needs is more "drive," or dynamism, or self-sacrifice, or "creativity." In a sort of ghastly simplicity we remove the organ and demand the function. We make men without chests and expect of them virtue and enterprise. We laugh at honour and are shocked to find traitors in our midst. We castrate and bid the geldings be fruitful.[2]

Throughout the course of this book, I have developed a novel argument in support of making physician-assisted suicide a legally and morally permissible option for terminally ill patients who are still capable of conscious consent. I have argued that such an option enhances our ability to secure informed consent and that we fail to see this because we are insufficiently attentive to the special dilemma that these patients face. In this final chapter, I explore the pedagogical implications of my approach to this sensitive topic. I am especially concerned that my existentially minded perspective could be confusing or even harmful in the classroom.

Future doctors, pharmacists, and other medical professionals must ordinarily balance a concern for a patient's values with a commitment to achieving just and fair outcomes for all. How, then, can we press upon future medical professionals the need to respect a patient's personal beliefs and values without concluding that ethical considerations are *merely subjective* in general? How can we balance the need for ethical justification with a deep respect for the personal nature of end-of-life dilemmas? In chapter 2, I claimed that the syllogistic and existential approaches to mortality are, in some respects, incommensurable and irreconcilable. But professors have a responsibility for conveying the significance of both standpoints: Future medical professionals must be able to make dispassionate and well-reasoned ethical judgments, but they must also take seriously the individual character of end-of-life dilemmas.

It is true that the argument for informed consent that I have consistently advanced throughout this discussion constitutes a sound policy reason for making PAS permissible. But I have also stressed the *limits* of scientific and ethical expertise and pointed out the ways in which our obsession with policy formulation often obscures the patient perspective. This view helps to deflate a false sense of scientific and ethical objectivity, but it might also lead to the undermining of a student's confidence in her need and ability to produce just and fair ethical reasoning. Further, in chapters 4 and 5, respectively, I gave an account of how the patient's perspective transforms even the most basic of concepts: how we think about killing and how we conceptualize suicide. So even if my thesis concerning informed consent holds as a compelling policy prescription, I readily admit that the tone of my reflections on ethics could give students the false impression that ethics is only ever personal. This is especially true when we already have a tendency to abstract from particular dilemmas (i.e., terminally ill patients consciously confronting mortality) and make general assumptions about the nature of values.

My concern is grounded in my own experience teaching end-of-life issues to future doctors and pharmacists. One of the best students whom I have ever taught asked to meet with me after class one day. He confessed that his excitement about becoming a doctor was starting to wane since he was only now seeing the depth of the dilemmas he would be asked to face in the future. Moreover, he no longer knew what to make of the various ethical theories we studied earlier in the semester, as they now seemed impotent in the face of these dilemmas. He felt that he had become, so to speak, a "man without a chest," whose moral compass had become unmoored by the specificity of patient dilemmas. At the same time, he knew full well that he would be expected to act ethically and to protect the integrity of medicine were he to become a physician.

In an effort to address these concerns, I first make more explicit the kind of ethical model that I have been intimating throughout my discussion of end-of-life dilemmas. Then I discuss the basic conflicts between this alternative ethical model and the policy-dominant models that characterize much of modern medical ethics. Finally, I reference two other common topics in medical ethics (debates over the origin of moral status and the arguments concerning the ethics of enhancement) in order to suggest how we can teach end-of-life dilemmas in a similarly careful and balanced way.

***

In his 1971 novel *Love in the Ruins*, Walker Percy tells the story of a Louisiana psychiatrist who has invented the ontological lapsometer. As "a stethoscope of the human soul,"[3] this device diagnoses maladies of the spirit, parses out the different layers of the self, and roots out the underlying problem. Interestingly, patients feel healed, like themselves again, after being treated with this new invention. Percy, however, deftly mocks the notion that modern science could diagnose and treat complex mental states by reducing them to their physical manifestations. He underscores the existential rather than physiological dimension of human problems. And he is skeptical that the supposed success of the lapsometer treatments could be justified in terms of maximizing human freedom and control over one's destiny.

The prominent medical ethicist Carl Elliott has credited this story with motivating his interest in enhancement technologies. For him, the enduring lesson of Percy's account is that there is a fundamental difference between treating a "patient with a problem, and a person with a predicament."[4] For Elliott, *Love in the Ruins* anticipates the rise of psychopharmacology, especially drugs like Prozac. These drugs had a virtually immediate and enormous effect on many patients, who often reported feeling more like *themselves* than ever before.

Such enhancement technologies raise interesting questions about the nature of scientific progress and the extent to which individuals can become self-determining, truly *themselves*, by consuming pills. While Percy's novel parodies a childlike faith in the progress of modern science, Elliot's own philosophical view is more nuanced. He sometimes sees himself as diagnosing the ethical issues raised by psychopharmacology and other enhancement technologies rather than presenting an argument about their use.[5]

Walker Percy and Carl Elliott are philosophical kindred spirits whose own influences are eerily similar: Percy was inspired by the existentialism of Søren Kierkegaard, while Elliott regards Ludwig Wittgenstein as a source of inspiration. At first glance, Kierkegaard and Wittgenstein appear to be unlikely philosophical allies. Wittgenstein was a hero of analytic philosophers of language who regarded metaphysical and religious claims as meaningless and therefore bogus. Kierkegaard, on the contrary, suggested that the subjective truth of religious faith could result in what he called a "teleological suspension of the ethical."[6] In other words, moral rules could be temporarily set aside in the pursuit of a higher religious calling, even though such a decision would seem absurd and irrational to an outside observer.

If the philosophical similarities between Kierkegaard and Wittgenstein have been largely obscured, it is a result of Wittgenstein's reception and not his own writings. In fact, we are presented with a curious historical analogy: As Percy is to Elliott, Kierkegaard is to Wittgenstein. Wittgenstein's biographer Ray Monk discusses the extent to which Wittgenstein was inspired by Kierkegaard.[7] He especially notes Wittgenstein's appreciation for the limits of ethical and religious language. What lies beyond our ability to articulate ethical concepts may properly be called "nonsense," but that does not mean that it is bogus or insignificant. Rather, the limits of language condemn us to communicate ethical and religious truths only indirectly.[8]

Consider Wittgenstein's reflections on one of Kierkegaard's most famous observations. Kierkegaard writes, "What good would it do me if truth stood before me, cold and naked, not caring whether I recognized her or not?"[9] Here Kierkegaard is rebelling against philosophers who attempt to construct entire systems based on logically derived truth claims. He views subjectivity as a kind of trump card against this conceited philosophical impulse. The most beautifully constructed abstract arguments are vitiated by a subject who remains unmoved by their logic. Wittgenstein echoes this sentiment in the following passage on religion:

> I believe that one of the things Christianity says is that sound doctrines are all useless. That you have to change your *life*. (Or the direction of your life.) It says that all wisdom is cold; and that you can no more use it for setting your life to rights than you can forge iron when it is *cold*. The point is that a sound doctrine need not *take hold* of you; you can follow it as you would a doctor's

> prescription.—But here you need something to move you and turn you in a new direction. . . . Wisdom is passionless. But faith by contrast is what Kierkegaard calls a *passion.*[10]

These two sets of historical and philosophical connections (between Percy and Elliott and between Kierkegaard and Wittgenstein) present us with an alternative to the modern predilection for principle-based models. They provide a useful rejoinder to any attempt to ground and justify the rules, policies, and procedures that govern end-of-life choices. Recall the distinction (outlined in chapter 2) between the syllogistic and existential account of personhood. Insofar as modern medical ethics involves an attempt to provide rational criteria for action, it must presuppose an account of the individual that sometimes fails to adequately regard the first-person standpoint. On the contrary, this alternative philosophical view takes seriously the first-person nature of experience. It refuses to dismiss this perspective as nonsense, even if it is outside the scope of scientific and modern ethical inquiry.

An account inspired by these unlikely historical analogies might serve to redirect ethical inquiry to the personal nature of experience and value-formation, as well as the limits of scientific and principle-based ethical insight. This approach would have three basic themes: 1) a shared hostility to blurring the distinction between individuals: philosophical inquiry should be regarded as a first-person activity or even as a way of life rather than as a special sort of rule following; 2) a concern for unmasking contradictions, moral hypocrisy, and self-righteousness: Kierkegaard focused on the delusions of supposed Christians in his day, whereas Wittgenstein reserved his most venomous criticism for academic philosophers; and 3) a view of philosophy as descriptive rather than normative: Philosophy is useful not when it attempts to logically derive moral claims but rather when it identifies abuses of language and rearranges our concepts so that we can see the world differently. It makes the familiar look strange.

The goal of this endeavor is twofold: 1) exposing internal inconsistencies in present practices for the sake of reforming them (or at least acknowledging their limitations) and 2) breaking the spell of one's own presuppositions for the sake of self-knowledge. As the French philosopher Michel de Montaigne writes, "Habit puts to sleep the eye of judgment."[11] If philosophy demands the cultivation of one's judgment, then the first step is not to be seduced by what is accepted based on habit alone. We are psychologically predisposed to all sorts of fallacious reasoning having to do with habit: confirmation bias, circular argumentation, appeals to authority, and so on. Although we can never overcome these tendencies completely, we should mitigate them whenever we can. The payoff is some degree of clear thinking, as well as some knowledge about ourselves and the society in which we live.

This is not to suggest that every claim requires the same degree of justification. Many social mores, for example, are innocuous. But end-of-life dilemmas set a high bar for justification, especially when a conscious, terminally ill patient makes a request that is deemed to be illicit. Nor is it to imply that philosophical critique is inherently devastating to present practices. When raised to the level of critical awareness, much of what we do probably meets the appropriate justificatory burden. Or, even if it does not, we might continue with the present practice after seeing it with fresh eyes.

Despite whatever "cold wisdom" might be found in modern ethical analysis, this alternative view is an attempt to articulate what gets obscured in the process. For example, the passion that Kierkegaard and Wittgenstein discuss is not equivalent to the pleasure that utilitarians attempt to quantify. Passion is tied to a personal attempt to change one's life, whereas pleasure in the utilitarian sense is the substance of a putatively correct ethical principle. This *passion* is a modern invocation of an ancient ethical imperative: to live an examined life and to consider philosophy itself as a way of life.[12] So this existential model of philosophy challenges us to take seriously the particularity of persons.[13]

But even if one accepts this alternative model of what makes philosophy valuable as well as limited, there is perhaps a steep pedagogical price to be paid. As soon as values are regarded as deeply personal and based on one's own conception of a good life (or a good death),[14] then it becomes difficult to convey to future medical professionals the need to *justify* the ethical norms with which they must operate. Ideals of justice and fairness presuppose that individuals are *not* radically individuated and that we can make judgments across a variety of cases and a wide range of experiences. I have already conceded the need for uniform standards in the vast majority of end-of-life cases. But how are students supposed to react to the claim that some specific dilemmas are irreducibly personal? Or to put the question differently, How do we avoid conflating in the minds of students a respect for a patient's personal values with the idea that values are *merely subjective*?

Much of this confusion stems from the fact that this existential model seems to conflict with the way in which modern medical ethics has developed. Open almost any standard introduction to medical ethics, and you might discover some equally subtle philosophical lessons as in the textbook that Lewis analyzed. The content of these lessons, however, is the *opposite* of those found in the elementary school textbook. The authors of the elementary textbook imply that judgments of value are utterly personal and subjective. Lewis deemed this to entail a specious form of relativism. But the concern about the standard introduction to medical ethics is that it conveys to students a false sense of objectivity and authority. Students might assume that they can learn to transcend their subjective standpoint and learn to make correct ethical decisions. They do so by applying the correct ethical principle and following the logic of the argument to its practical conclusion.[15]

As a species of applied ethics, medical ethics is the kind of discipline that frequently moves from theory to practice. In other words, students often learn about competing theories of right and wrong, and then they apply these principles to specific cases.[16] But beginning a class by discussing how ethical theories are constructed and evaluated puts a certain understanding of medical ethics at the forefront of a student's mind. And structuring an introductory textbook in this way makes the practice of ethics seem like a matter of theoretical evaluation and application. The implied philosophical lesson is that there is some ethical wisdom being brought to bear upon seemingly intractable dilemmas.

As Lewis notes, the subtle lesson in the elementary school textbook is self-defeating: It undermines a student's ability to make strong claims to truth, even as we continue to expect that of rational adults. It cultivates a deep and serious form of hypocrisy, whereby students learn to falsely disavow their beliefs even as they genuinely affirm them. In the context of medical ethics, we are sometimes hypocrites in the opposite sense: We give students the impression that they are gaining expertise, even as we also hope that they will be sensitive to the deeply personal nature of values. This is especially true when it comes to grappling with end-of-life dilemmas.

If this is so, then these dilemmas provide a strange and singular exception to Lewis's argument about inculcating virtue. Under normal conditions, the relativism that angers Lewis is indeed a genuine threat to education. Yet in these specific cases, the virtuous doctor is the one who recognizes her own biases and lack of expertise. How can this mixed message be adequately conveyed to future medical professionals? In other words, how can professors walk the fine line between equipping students with the tools for making sound ethical judgments while also insisting that some dilemmas are existentially exceptional? Students should not leave an ethics class with a false sense of expertise. But I am also worried that they might leave the class having their own moral confidence undermined. All things being equal, the students who experience this sense of crisis might become the most sensitive and thoughtful future doctors. What obligations, if any, do professors have toward their students when discussing such delicate issues?

***

There are surprisingly few reflections on the nature of modern medical ethics. Much of the work being done in this field takes for granted the idea that we could codify some principles to help us make more rational decisions.[17] In this way, modern medical ethics has become increasingly legalistic over the past few decades. But whether this conception of ethics makes sense or not is seldom raised. Scholars sometimes engage in a metadebate over the meaning, purpose, and value of this discipline, but these projects are few and far between. Occasionally someone raises the question of whether medical ethics is even something new unto itself. Onora O'Neill, for instance, argues, "Bioethics is not a discipline, nor even a new discipline; I doubt whether it will ever be a discipline. It has become a meeting ground for a number of disciplines, discourses, and organizations concerned with the ethical, legal, and social questions raised by advances in medicine, science, and biotechnology."[18]

Other scholars identify the complicated relationship between medical ethics scholarship and medical ethics advocacy. Daniel Wikler writes, "Bioethics has had a dual character; it is a field of inquiry, with characteristic methods, and also a particular kind of advocacy. Those roles do not necessarily jibe."[19] Wikler's point is that patient advocates are not free to question certain practices like informed consent, whereas scholars remain uncommitted to such presuppositions.

The fact that modern medical ethics often adopts a legalistic approach to ethical dilemmas is a contingent fact about its historical development. Whether it is something distinct or not, it is old enough to be critically evaluated but young enough to be open to reform. It is true that philosophy of medicine is ancient, and versions of ethical codes in the United States have been around for well over a century and a half.[20] Also, there are many ways of identifying the contemporary origins of medical ethics. However, I think that the best way of dating the beginning of this new discipline (if it is one) is to focus on the 1949 Nuremberg Code.[21]

I would defend this time line for two distinct reasons: First, the Nuremberg Code emphasizes the idea of informed consent. To my mind, this is the most significant ethical advance of the twentieth century. The requirement it imposes far exceeds the logic of nonmaleficence. It brings ontological and epistemological issues to the forefront. How do we circumscribe the boundaries of the self in order to determine whether a patient is making an autonomous decision? How informed must informed consent be, and how can doctors figure this out? Later ethical codes, like the Declaration of Helsinki and the Belmont Report, expand on the insights of the Nuremberg Code, but this document raised the most significant ethical issue of our time. The rise of institutional review boards and hospital ethics committees would later take place in its wake.

The second reason this is a good place to start is because of the atrocity to which the Nuremberg Code responded. Modern medical ethics was arguably founded as a reaction to the unfathomable harm that can be imposed on individuals when researchers have no ethical regard for their lives. In her criticism of how medical ethics has been transformed over the years, Rachel Haliburton discusses these heroic origins.[22] She does this in order to contrast the current state of affairs of medical ethics with its original mandate. As I have already claimed, our current ethical analysis of end-of-life dilemmas does not sufficiently protect individual patients and their personal values in some cases. It fails to take personhood, consciousness, and consent seriously. So it is useful to observe how medical ethics has evolved (for better or worse) over the past seventy years. A new discipline emerged to protect individuals against the encroachment of scientific power and authority. But as I have also consistently argued, in its current manifestation, medical ethics often corroborates rather than challenges the very authority it was designed to check.

Another way in which medical ethics has drastically changed is by becoming a popular and institutionally recognized specialization in philosophy. It is now possible to serve on a hospital ethics committee, to pursue a PhD in bioethics, and to instruct the next generation of doctors and nurses in the ethics of their future profession. In this way, medical ethics provides a new and exciting avenue for becoming a public intellectual. It provides philosophers with a ready-made response to the accusation that they engage in armchair speculation. As a practical and applied discipline, it offers a way for them to rappel out of the ivory tower. Further, its dilemmas are omnipresent and immediately recognizable to anyone who has lived long enough to be personally confronted by them. Innovative teachers can contrive compelling but fictitious examples pertaining to trolleys and lifeboats, but medical ethics deals with reality as such.[23]

For these reasons, an often-maligned but ancient discipline gains credibility when it can demonstrate its usefulness in the modern world. The partnership between science, law, and ethics is beneficial for all parties.[24] Science as a descriptive discipline gains normative support for its claims. Laws governing end-of-life dilemmas are seen as ethically sound instead of merely imposed as authoritative.

Moreover, there are good philosophical and prudential reasons for the typical structure of an introductory textbook. One good philosophical reason is that students need to have some command of ethical theory before they can delve into specific cases. Theories can serve as frameworks and guidelines for thinking. Students might stumble along in the dark if they do not have some theoretical tools for considering hard cases. They might make decisions in a random or ad hoc manner.

There are two additional prudential reasons for structuring a textbook in this way. First, distinguishing sharply between theory and practice makes it easier for the professor to fully discuss both of these elements of an ethical decision. It is possible to distribute the discussion of ethical theory throughout the course. However, this would likely muddy the waters instead of providing students with a sharp contrast between ethical views like deontology and utilitarianism. For instance, one could jump immediately into hard cases and allow the details of utilitarianism to emerge in the course of conversation. But this is not likely to give students a strong enough theoretical foundation for making decisions.

The second prudential reason is to capitalize on the institutional credibility that medical ethics offers to philosophy. The academic turf that has been conceded to philosophy would be squandered if medical ethics were taught as a "best practices" kind of course. In other words, anyone who can comprehend and convey the principles found in the Belmont Report could teach students the prevailing legal and moral norms that govern medical research. Philosophers have been given a golden opportunity to prove that they can contribute some unique expertise. It is no wonder that introductory courses often begin with a discussion, for instance, on deontological principles. Whether the imposition of a technical vocabulary helps or hinders learning is, I think, an open question. But the fact that it is used is understandable, given the historical conditions under which medical ethics developed.

There are many problems with teaching an introductory course in this way, however. Students might get the impression that ethics occupies its own theoretical domain and that ethicists bring to bear some unique expertise. This is not to deny that expertise could take the form of an ability to ask timely and pointed questions or to compare and contrast different claims about what is morally right. But the notion that ethical expertise could take the form of propositional knowledge is doubtful at best. My concern is that students might form this conclusion if the professor is not careful.

It is easy to see why ethical expertise cannot be described in this way. The arguments against this line of thinking are ancient, going back to what the Pyrrhonian skeptics called "the problem of the criterion."[25] There are many versions of this influential argument, and it has proven to be especially important for contemporary epistemology.[26] For our purposes, it stresses the fact that no claim to truth could ever be self-justifying. In order to defend the truth of any proposition, one must always appeal to an external standard. But then that standard will also require the same defense, and so on. So justification becomes an infinite regress. For this reason, being an expert in applying a utilitarian calculus does not mean that one can defend the truth of utilitarianism itself. So if a student believes that she has learned a new and magical secret about how to tell right from wrong, this does not mean that she is able to justify using that principle instead of another.

An obvious way of mitigating this pedagogical danger is to remind students that theories have to fit our considered judgments about what it right and true. In other words, if I devise an ethical theory that seems beautifully coherent, it must also seem plausible to people who would put it into practice. Otherwise, we would have reason to doubt whether it was true at all. Sometimes this is explained by appealing to the idea of "reflective equilibrium."[27] General principles must be balanced against the facts of particular cases; theoretical claims must be weighed against conventional practices and beliefs. In this way, both our moral theories and our typical practices are always subject to reform and refinement.

Under normal circumstances, it makes sense to say that ethics involves the training of one's judgment in order to carefully weigh and balance theory and practice. But there is a glaring problem with adopting this approach in the context of end-of-life dilemmas. On my view, these situations do not provide the necessary ingredients in order for an ethicist to work in this way. Throughout this book, I have maintained that end-of-life dilemmas are existential outliers. The values that a patient expresses when confronting her own mortality are not standard candidates for ethical understanding and evaluation. It is true that the patient must be deemed competent, but this does not give doctors or proxies license to claim what they want about her mental state. Nor does it mean that they must endorse whatever difficult decision she makes afterward. The patient faces a devil's choice between different types of death, not a decision about whether to live or die.

Here is an example of how reflective equilibrium breaks down when applied to end-of-life situations. Whenever I teach this concept, I tell my students about the time I had to travel from Atlanta, Georgia, to Greenville, South Carolina. I had no idea where in the state Greenville was located, nor did I have any idea of how to get to my friend's house once I arrived in the city. So I needed two different maps in order to get to my destination. The virtue of the state map was its clarity, but it lacked the details I needed to find the house. The city map had all the details I needed, but the view was no longer clear. There was too much information and not enough perspective. Both of these maps were necessary; one could not be superimposed upon the other and still help me navigate.

By analogy, theories provide us with a view from above, while particular cases and present practices give us a view on the ground. In this way, we can have both a clear perspective and detailed understanding but not at the same time. We exercise our ethical judgment when we zoom in and out, reforming and refining along the way. This is what it means to use reflective equilibrium in the course of making an ordinary ethical judgment.

But the problem with end-of-life dilemmas is that we have no view on the ground. There is no map to guide us there. For example, our ethical principles have equipped us to have abstract conversations about suicide. As I have argued, this has only led to a false equivalence that ignores relevant differences in context. Provided that the patient is both terminally ill and competent, we do not need to share her values, and we certainly cannot stand in her shoes. In almost any other situation that a doctor could confront, patients can be reasonably substituted for one another. Organisms are interchangeable. But that is simply not the case here.

So even if we move beyond a superficial understanding of theory and practice, we face another pedagogical challenge. How can we avoid alienating smart and sensitive students who begin to understand the gravity of end-of-life situations? One student might defend physician-assisted suicide on the grounds that it achieves some utilitarian goals. He might view his analysis as being not merely insightful but also morally correct. Another student might realize that this approach to ethics has met its match in end-of-life dilemmas. She finds that she cannot meaningfully use reflective equilibrium to resolve this problem. Further, she might be wary of finding herself involved both personally and professionally in these situations. All things being equal, the students who feel this most deeply might be the best but also the most reluctant future doctors.

It is easy to say that philosophy professors are obligated only to truth rather than practical issues, like professional development. But this is as shortsighted as assuming that one can teach Nietzsche to first-year theology students without considering the audience. There must be some consideration for the mental and emotional state of one's students, whether their religious faith or their faith in medicine is being tested. And even if the smart and sensitive students decide to push through and accept the burden of dealing with end-of-life dilemmas, they will be expected to adhere to best practices and hospital regulations. Their philosophical concerns might strike their colleagues as idle or even self-indulgent chatter.

Moreover, some patients and their families might be only too willing to defer to the supposed judgment and expertise of the doctor. They could genuinely believe that scientific and ethical expertise are somehow related. They could be conflating the two without knowing it. Or they could simply be wishing for a way to abdicate the moral responsibility that they have toward themselves or their loved ones. It is not hard to imagine someone terrified of pulling the plug on a loved one and looking for any indication from the doctor about the right course of action. Regardless of the reasons behind the belief, the doctor could still be regarded by others as a putative ethical authority. This is true even if she absolutely refuses to think of herself in this way.

Just as there are institutional constraints on our future doctor, there is also pressure on our hypothetical professor. It might be difficult to explain the pedagogical significance of a medical ethics course if the outcome of its deliberations is indefinite. A discipline based on a thoughtful recognition of its own limits might seem overly "meta" or even idiosyncratic or elitist. The contrast between this attitude and the historical conditions under which the discipline was born could not be starker: There was a profound need for an ethical check on scientific encroachment, and this was accomplished through the formulation of principles and best practices. To deny that this is what makes ethics important seems like a voluntary surrender of recognition, respect, and institutional credibility.

Ethics could still be regarded as a first-person activity. So the alternative conception of ethics that I have discussed throughout this book could still obtain. In this case, the professor serves as a kind of Socratic midwife for the students, each of whom is learning to think for herself. But no matter how true and honest this approach to ethics might be, it either downplays or explicitly rejects what made medical ethics possible (and necessary) in the first place.

I think that professors of medical ethics have a serious obligation to do their best to leave students with a nuanced view of end-of-life situations. This involves educating them about the best practices that they will need to know. But it also means stressing the limits of what they can reasonably claim, both scientifically and ethically. It might also include passing down this duty to educate: Our future doctor might have to take the time to explain to her patients or her patients' families the limits of her expertise.

If we view ethical principles as valuable heuristic devices, then we can meaningfully incorporate them into a course in medical ethics. Equipping future medical professionals with analytic tools need not involve convincing them of the absolute truth of any particular theoretical perspective. Likewise, inculcating a sensitivity to the personal character of end-of-life dilemmas does not need to collapse into moral relativism. *These end-of-life beliefs and values are rationally intelligible, even if they are also personal.* Future doctors need to hone their ability to recognize the legitimacy of beliefs and values that they do not happen to hold personally.

***

In this final section, I explore some other topics in medical ethics where this alternative existential model clearly applies (e.g., debates over the origin of moral status and conflicts concerning enhancement technologies). End-of-life issues, on the contrary, are not often recognized as ambiguous in the same way and to the same degree. This is true even though they are just as philosophically befuddling as debates in these other domains. So although it may be difficult to achieve an appropriate pedagogical balance with respect to end-of-life dilemmas, I think that we can improve our ability to do so by considering how we might already teach other controversial topics.

The lively moral and political debates over the origin of moral status and the ethics of enhancement technologies are ripe for this kind of existential analysis. What makes these issues philosophically interesting is our *failure* to attain consensus through the formulation of rational principles. These issues are rife with conceptual ambiguity, abuses of language, deep epistemological questions, and intractable ontological disputes about the boundaries of the self. For these reasons, these topics could serve as models for how to teach end-of-life issues to future medical professionals.

Take, for instance, the quagmire of the modern abortion debate. Calling this dispute a debate is already an abuse of language, as there is no common agreement on underlying first principles. What we require in order to render a verdict on the question of abortion is a nonarbitrary way of determining the origin of moral status. But we cannot agree on the necessary and sufficient conditions for determining this. A pro-life critic of abortion might even regard the question itself as meaningless, as moral status does not need to be "determined" after conception has taken place. While a pro-life advocate might insist that conception is the obvious origin of moral status, an author who defends the moral and legal permissibility of abortion might object that a person is not yet present in the moral sense.[28]

One might have good reason for believing that consciousness is central to personhood, but how would one demonstrate this to a pro-life advocate? Conversely, one might have good reason for adopting conception as a nonarbitrary starting point for moral status, but how could this ever be demonstrated to someone who sees only a clump of cells at this stage? One way to justify either claim might be to appeal to empirical evidence. However, we cannot even agree on what would *count* as empirical evidence in this case. Pointing at cells on a sonogram does not settle the conceptual question of what moral status those cells have. And even to call them "cells" is already to frame the debate in a misleading way, according to the pro-life advocate.[29]

A seemingly simple term like *potential*[30] can be given several radically different interpretations. So, too, can the idea that there is a time line of human development "from zygote to irreversible coma."[31] No one would deny that there are different phases of life, but we cannot agree on which of those stages deserves moral protection. One basic point of contention is whether personhood is required for moral standing over and above the biological existence of an organism.

Appealing to biological existence as a baseline criterion for moral status only raises new questions. Jeff McMahan rejects this idea, arguing that human beings are not organisms but rather persons whose consciousness is morally significant. Setting aside questions about the possibility of disembodied consciousness, an organism is a necessary but not sufficient condition for moral status. But even if this claim were to be rejected, McMahan presents a separate argument to show how six-day-old embryos are not organisms either. He argues that these cells are like "marbles in a sack," completely lacking the differentiation and specialized function required for counting something as an organism.[32] Cells that are not organized in any meaningful way have human DNA, but they do not rise to the level of organisms, much less persons.

Debates over the origin of moral status often have the merit of bringing all of this conceptual ambiguity to the forefront. Perhaps treating one's own premises as self-evident is not a naïve and mistaken attempt to justify them but rather a rhetorical strategy for berating an interlocutor into recognizing what should be clear. This strategy might stem from the recognition that there is no absolute way to rationally demonstrate the necessary and sufficient criteria for moral status. These intellectual skirmishes often revolve around competing claims about appropriate rules, policies, and procedures. But a different way of analyzing these arguments rejects this method in favor of a close description of clashing presuppositions. Pointing out inconsistency and incoherence might not ever lead to the establishment of a more rational governing principle. If it does, then it will have succeeded only provisionally. This kind of immanent critique depends solely upon a clear description of one's assumptions and commitments. It neither constructs nor discovers a more rational principle *on its own.*

In the same way, studying specific end-of-life dilemmas could have the same pedagogical outcomes. On my view, not recognizing the legitimacy of PAS constitutes a failure to adequately account for one's own commitments (especially concerning informed consent). If this kind of philosophical critique leads only to thoughtful self-examination and the training of one's judgment, then maybe that is all we can hope for. Further, it seems valuable to recognize the role that a conceptual framework plays in our ability to even describe the dilemma. This suggests an interesting parallel between determining the origin of moral status and determining its end. When we ask the question "When does life begin?" what we really mean is "When does moral status obtain?" I suppose that we could ask whether a zygote is "alive" in the same sense as an organism, but the context for that question never seems to be purely scientific.

We often seem to understand this in the context of debates over the origin of moral status. But when it comes to end-of-life debates, we suddenly defer to a misplaced sense of scientific and ethical authority. Too often we fail to have the kinds of informed conversations about the relationship between persons and organisms and about the effects of superpharmaceuticals. We use terms like *killing* and *suicide* without honestly confronting their complexity in some end-of-life dilemmas. Why should the question of moral status be so difficult to resolve in one context but so easy to resolve in another?

This disparity is also evident when we compare end-of-life issues with arguments concerning the ethics of enhancement. So here again, we might gain some insight into how best to approach end-of-life debates pedagogically. My favorite example of a controversial medical intervention is the one I mentioned earlier in this chapter: the use of Prozac to treat depression. Peter Kramer's book *Listening to Prozac* encapsulates many of the conceptual issues inherent in discussions over psychopharmacology. One of his patients, a woman named Tess, experienced an extraordinary transformation while on this drug. Her symptoms were first treated by an older antidepressant called imipramine. Kramer decided that Tess's symptoms were not being adequately managed by this drug on account of the way she sobbed uncontrollably when reminded of an ex-lover. Prozac fully suppressed these symptoms, but it also did much more. The wallflower morphed into a social butterfly, and the adequately performing worker successfully competed for a major promotion.

Kramer wonders whether his intervention has transgressed the boundaries of medicine, transforming rather than restoring his patient. If the purpose of medicine is to heal, then something akin to (but perhaps better than) imipramine would be sufficient. Prozac might be classified as a different drug entirely since its effects (at least on this particular patient) seemed categorically different from antidepressants. Kramer wondered, too, how to draw the line between legitimate psychopharmacology and other mind-altering but illicit substances.[33] In spite of his concerns about the limits of medicine and the social implications of medicating sad people, Kramer continued to prescribe the drug to Tess. In large part, this was because Tess reported that she did not feel like herself when she was briefly off the pills. This observation confounded Kramer: Based on this logic, Tess had only briefly been *herself* in her entire life!

Two observers could study a fetus and draw opposite conclusions about its moral status. Likewise, two observers could reach different conclusions after examining Tess's transformation and her claim about her own self-identity. Since depression leads to deficient functioning, it would make sense to argue that a person whose symptoms have been treated can now live as she *would have* were it not for her condition. On the other hand, this kind of counterfactual claim seems suspicious when the transformation is so extreme. A third observer might not care whether the improvement is authentic in any way. It is self-evident that Tess's mood improved, and maybe that trumps any ethical concerns about her use of Prozac.

One of Kramer's most persistent critics, Carol Freedman, is concerned about both the ethics and the efficacy of prescribing a drug that radically transforms a personality. She finds it disturbing that a drug could have such an immediate and profound effect on something as personal as one's self-identity. In her article "Aspirin for the Mind? Some Ethical Worries about Psychopharmacology," Freedman distinguishes between a rational cause and a mechanical cause of one's behavior.[34] These are two different descriptions of the same phenomenon.[35]

Rational causes emanate from a *self* with its reasons, justified or not, for acting a certain way. Mechanical causes describe human behavior as a manifestation of a biological state. Both descriptions can be true simultaneously. If I ask why you were sad yesterday, you might tell me that you were fired from your job. It could also be true that the serotonin levels in your brain were outside of their normal range.

Freedman worries about the fact that Prozac so effectively transformed Tess's personality. Set aside any consideration about whether it should count as medicine. The bare fact that it had such an immediate impact "makes it too easy for us to see ourselves in mechanistic terms. In this sense it jeopardizes our dignity as responsible persons who owe it to ourselves to struggle toward insight through dialogue."[36] Whether Prozac was an effective form of treatment for Tess depends upon what that requires. It is true that her mood improved astonishingly and that genuinely good things happened in her life. However, she never bothered to rationally understand the root causes of her problem. Lacking this insight means, for Freedman at least, that Kramer simply put a Band-Aid on a festering wound. If happiness is more than simply feeling good in the present moment, then Kramer has elected to "fix" the organism rather than the person.

Here, as in the case of determining the origin of moral status, we see important questions concerning personhood and moral status at the forefront of the debate. But in the context of debates over physician-assisted suicide and continuous sedation until death, we do not typically notice the same sort of concerns. These other topics also challenge us to confront conceptual ambiguity. For instance, since medicine is supposed to cure or restore but not transform, Prozac seemed categorically different from the antidepressant imipramine. What are we to make, then, of drugs that neither restore nor transform but rather slowly eradicate consciousness? And why is it that we do not see this question asked more often in debates over end-of-life dilemmas?

There is no doubt that most uses of morphine and its pharmaceutical cousins fall within the scope of medicine. But perhaps palliation is as different from CSD as imipramine is from Prozac.[37] This illuminates something about the status of the self and the difficulty in defining a medical intervention. Patients need palliative care, just as a patient might need an antidepressant to treat symptoms. It is even true that a patient could require CSD to alleviate intractable pain. However, she might be in that situation because she did not have access to PAS six months earlier. And the way in which we alleviate the symptoms is by rendering her continuously unconscious until her organism dies.

Dr. Kramer alleviated Tess's symptoms by reducing her problems to a mechanical, not rational, causal explanation. In other words, he "fixed" her organism without regard for whether she rationally understood the reasons behind her depression. Consequently, Tess has undergone an absurd loss of self: Her doctor has enabled her to view herself as a finely tuned organism rather than a rational and self-conscious agent. Even as she reports feeling more like herself than ever before, it is the *feeling* and not the understanding of her condition that she prizes.

We have treated end-of-life dilemmas in a similar way but with one disturbing twist: The patient is compelled to consent to self-eradication and the continued existence of the organism. The way in which a patient copes with her depression or with her impending mortality gets reduced to a series of treatable physiological symptoms. In both cases, a uniform and pseudoempirical solution gets imposed upon a complex problem. The status of the organism (and not the person) becomes the key criterion for defining when a patient is dead and what counts as medicine. Curing becomes transforming, and treatment morphs into annihilation. In either case, the patient does not survive the cure.

But enough talk. Let us bring it back to the beginning and give Seneca the last word: "Put aside the studies which you have pursued throughout your life; Death will deliver the final judgment in your case. This is what I mean: your debates and learned talks, your maxims gathered from the teachings of the wise, your cultured conversation,—all these afford no proof of the real strength of your soul. Even the most timid man can deliver a bold speech."[38]

NOTES

1. C. S. Lewis, "Men without Chests," in *The Abolition of Man* (New York: HarperOne, 2015), 2.
2. Lewis, "Men without Chests," 26.
3. Walker Percy, *Love in the Ruins* (New York: Picador, 1999), 62.
4. See Michael Szpir, "An interview with Carl Elliott," accessed February 15, 2015, http://www.americanscientist.org/bookshelf/pub/carl-elliott.
5. For a good example of Elliott's balanced approached to tough ethical issues, see Carl Elliott, "Amputees by Choice," in *Better Than Well: American Medicine Meets the American Dream* (New York: W. W. Norton, 2003).
6. This concept is central to Kierkegaard's view of Abraham in *Fear and Trembling*, trans. Alastair Hannay (London: Penguin Classics, 1986).
7. Ray Monk, *Ludwig Wittgenstein: The Duty of Genius* (New York: Penguin Books, 1991).
8. This is the main theme of Wittgenstein's *Lecture on Ethics*, November 1929, accessed May 30, 2015, http://sackett.net/WittgensteinEthics.pdf.
9. Søren Kierkegaard, *The Journals of Kierkegaard*, trans. Alexander Dru (New York: Harper & Row, 1959), 44–45.
10. Monk, *Ludwig Wittgenstein*, 490.
11. Michel de Montaigne, "Of Custom," *Essays of Montaigne*, vol. 1, trans. Charles Cotton, accessed August 15, 2016, http://oll.libertyfund.org/titles/montaigne-essays-of-montaigne-vol-1.
12. To see how the idea of philosophy as a way of life unifies ancient and modern thought, I would recommend Pierre Hadot, *Philosophy as a Way of Life: Spiritual Exercises from Socrates to Foucault* (Malden, MA: Wiley-Blackwell, 1995).
13. In chapter 2, I pointed out how the difficulty in doing this is built into our very language.
14. To clarify, I have not claimed (and do not think) that the *content* of a patient's end-of-life preferences must be grounded in any particular conception of the good life. On my view, there is no morally appropriate way to confront one's own imminent demise.
15. I understand that virtue ethics has becomes a mainstream counterpoint to a theory-based or principle-based approach. But if the virtue ethicist refuses to give any content to his injunction to act virtuously, then I wonder whether virtue ethics is subject to the same sort of criticism as the model that I have used throughout this book. On the other hand, if virtue ethics attempts to spell out *what makes* an action virtuous, then it arguably starts to look like just another principle-based model.
16. This is not an indictment of *all* modern medical ethics, but I think it is uncontroversial to point out this prevalent tendency (especially in introductory classes).

17. See Rosamond Rhodes, "Understanding the Trusted Doctor and Constructing a Theory of Bioethics," *Theoretical Medicine* 22 (2001): 493–504.
18. Onora O'Neill, *Autonomy and Trust in Bioethics* (Cambridge: Cambridge University Press, 2002), 1.
19. Daniel Wikler, "What Has Bioethics to Offer Health Policy?" *Millbank Quarterly* 69, no. 2 (1991): 236.
20. The first code of ethics of the American Medical Association was introduced in 1847.
21. See Nuremberg Code, "Trials of War Criminals before the Nuremberg Military Tribunals under Control Council Law No. 10," vol. 2 (Washington, DC: U.S. Government Printing Office 1949), 181–82.
22. Rachel Haliburton, *Autonomy and the Situated Self: A Challenge to Bioethics* (Lanham, MD: Lexington Books, 2014).
23. Based on a 1967 thought experiment by Philippa Foot, "the trolley problem" has recently become a popular ethical dilemma to explore. For a colloquial discussion of its main themes, consider Thomas Cathcart, *The Trolley Problem: Or Would You Throw the Fat Guy Off the Bridge?* (New York: Workman, 2013).
24. Recall the collaborative effort to construct the Uniform Determination of Death Act.
25. In the following passage, Sextus Empiricus discusses "the reciprocal mode," which is one of the many weapons that a skeptic can use to cut down an argument: "For a proof always requires a standard in order to be confirmed, and a standard always requires a proof in order to be shown to be true. A proof cannot be sound if there is no standard there already, nor can a standard be true if a proof has not already been made convincing." Sextus Empiricus, *Outlines of Skepticism*, ed. Julia Annas and Jonathan Barnes (Cambridge: Cambridge University Press, 2000), 1:114.
26. See especially R. M. Chisholm, *The Problem of the Criterion* (Milwaukee: Marquette University Press, 1973).
27. This concept plays an important role in John Rawls's entire corpus. See John Rawls, "Outline of a Decision Procedure for Ethics," *Philosophical Review* 60, no. 2 (1951): 177–97.
28. See, for instance, Mary Anne Warren, "On the Moral and Legal Status of Abortion," *Monist* 57, no. 1 (January 1973): 43–61. She argues that five criteria are central to the idea of personhood, including consciousness, reasoning, self-motivated activity, the capacity to communicate, and a sense of self-awareness.
29. The dilemma we face here seems like the secular equivalent of analyzing the Catholic belief about the Eucharist. Putting a consecrated host under a microscope does not prove that it is simply bread, just as pointing at a fertilized egg in a petri dish does not prove that it is merely a clump of cells.
30. See Don Marquis, "Why Abortion is Immoral," *Journal of Philosophy* 86 (April 1989): 183–202. Here he argues that a fetus has a "future like ours." To deprive it of this future is wrong for the same reason that killing an adult human being is wrong. Also see the President's Council on Bioethics' argument about the "immanent potentiality" of an IVF embryo: "An embryo is, by definition and by its nature, potentially a fully developed human person; its potential for maturation is a characteristic it *actually* has, and from the start. . . . A bird forced to live in a cage its entire life may never learn to fly. But this does not mean it is less of a bird, or that it lacks the immanent potentiality to fly on feathered wings. It means only that a caged bird—like an in vitro human embryo—has been deprived of its proper environment." President's Council on Bioethics, "Human Cloning and Human Dignity: An Ethical Inquiry," in *Biomedical Ethics*, ed. David DeGrazia et al. (New York: McGraw-Hill, 2011): 516–17.
31. President's Council on Bioethics, "Human Cloning," 515.
32. Jeff McMahan argues this point in "Killing Embryos for Stem Cell Research," *Metaphilosophy* 38, nos. 2–3 (2007): 178–83.
33. Peter Kramer, *Listening to Prozac: A Psychiatrist Explores Antidepressant Drugs and the Remaking of the Self*, rev. ed. (New York: Penguin Books, 1997).
34. Carol Freedman, "Aspirin for the Mind? Some Ethical Worries about Psychopharmacology," in *Enhancing Human Traits: Ethical and Social Implications*, ed. Erik Parens (Washington, DC: Georgetown University Press, 1998).

35. Recall the discussion in chapter 4 of the difference between rational accounts and material explanations.
36. Freedman, "Aspirin for the Mind?" 145.
37. I realize that enhancement and eradication are different outcomes, but I am strictly making a point about how to define a medical intervention.
38. Lucius Annaeus Seneca, *Moral Epistles*, trans. Richard M. Gummere, in the *Loeb Classical Library* 75 (Cambridge: Harvard University Press, 1917), vol. 4, epistle 26.

Bibliography

Ackerman, Terrence F. "Why Doctors Should Intervene." *Hastings Center Report* 12 (1982): 14–17.

American Medical Association. *Code of Ethics*, Section 5.6. "Sedation to Unconsciousness in End-of-Life Care" (2016). Accessed March 3, 2015. http://www.ama-assn.org/ama/pub/physician-resources/medical-ethics/code-medical-ethics.page.

———. "Ethical Opinion E-2.06: Capital Punishment." In *Code of Medical Ethics of the American Medical Association* (Chicago: American Medical Association, 2006): 19–20.

Barbash, Fred. "After 18 Botched IV Attempts on a Screaming, Bleeding Inmate, Ohio Gets Another Chance to Execute Him." *Washington Post*. March 17, 2016. Accessed August 1, 2016. https://www.washingtonpost.com/news/morning-mix/wp/2016/03/17/after-18-botched-iv-attempts-on-a-screaming-bleeding-inmate-ohio-gets-another-chance-to-execute-him/.

Bartels, Stephen J., and John A. Naslund. "The Underside of the Silver Tsunami—Older Adults and Mental Health Care." *New England Journal of Medicine* 368 (2013): 493–96.

Battin, Margaret P. "Terminal Sedation: Pulling the Sheet over Our Eyes." *Hastings Center Report* 38, no. 5 (2008): 27–30.

Becker, Jo, and Scott Shane. "Secret 'Kill List' Proves a Test of Obama's Principles and Will. *New York Times*, May 29, 2012. Accessed June 2, 2014. http://www.nytimes.com/2012/05/29/world/obamas-leadership-in-war-on-al-qaeda.html.

Bellow, Jason. "New: 87 Deceased NFL Players Test Positive for Brain Disease." *Frontline*. September 18, 2015. Accessed June 1, 2016. http://www.pbs.org/wgbh/frontline/article/new-87-deceased-nfl-players-test-positive-for-brain-disease/.

Bernacki, Rachelle E., and Susan D. Block. "Communication about Serious Illness Care Goals: A Review and Synthesis of Best Practices." *JAMA Internal Medicine* 174, no.12 (December 2014): 1994–2003.

Bernat, James. "The Whole-Brain Concept of Death Remains Optimum Public Policy." *Journal of Law, Medicine, and Ethics* 34, no. 1 (2006): 35–43.

Bernat, James L., Bernard Gert, and R. Peter Mogielnicki. "Patient Refusal of Hydration and Nutrition: An Alternative to Physician-Assisted Suicide or Voluntary Active Euthanasia." *Archives of Internal Medicine* 153 (December 1993): 2723–28.

Bouvia v. Superior Court, 225 Cal Rpt. 297 (Cal. App 2d Dist 1986).

Burgess, Anthony. *A Clockwork Orange*. New York: W. W. Norton, 1995.

Burkeman, Oliver. "Why can't the World's Greatest Minds Solve the Mystery of Consciousness?" January 21, 2015. Accessed November 1, 2015. https://www.theguardian.com/science/2015/jan/21/-sp-why-cant-worlds-greatest-minds-solve-mystery-consciousness.

Callahan, Daniel. "Killing and Allowing to Die." *Hastings Center Report* 19, special supplement (1989): 5–6.

———. "When Self-Determination Runs Amok." *Hastings Center Report* 22, no. 2 (1992): 52–55.

Caplan, Arthur, James McCartney, and Dominic Sisti, eds. *The Case of Terri Schiavo: Ethics at the End of Life*. New York: Prometheus Books, 2006.

Cathcart, Thomas. *The Trolley Problem: Or Would You Throw the Fat Guy Off the Bridge?* New York: Workman, 2013.

Chalmers, David J. "Facing Up to the Problem of Consciousness." *Journal of Consciousness Studies* 2, no. 3 (1995): 200–19.

Chisholm, R. M. *The Problem of the Criterion*. Milwaukee: Marquette University Press, 1973.

Cholbi, Michael. "No Last Resort: Pitting the Right to Die against the Right to Medical Self-Determination." *Journal of Ethics: An International Philosophical Review* 19 (2015): 143–57.

Churchland, Patricia. *Braintrust: What Neuroscience Tells Us about Morality*. Princeton: Princeton University Press, 2011.

Churchland, Paul M. "Eliminative Materialism and the Propositional Attitudes." *Journal of Philosophy* (1981): 67–90.

Cleveland Clinic. "The Power of Every One." *Centennial Campaign*. Accessed June 16, 2015. http://giving.clevelandclinic.org/articles/power-every-one.

"Correspondence." *New England Journal of Medicine* 324 (1991): 561–62.

DeGrazia, David, and Thomas Mappes. *Biomedical Ethics*. New York: McGraw-Hill, 2011.

Descartes, René. *Meditations on First Philosophy*. In *Discourse on Method and Meditations on First Philosophy*. Translated by Donald Cress. Indianapolis: Hackett, 1998.

Doerflinger, Richard M., and Carlos Gomez. "Killing the Pain Not the Patient: Palliative Care vs. Assisted Suicide." *United States Conference of Catholic Bishops*. Accessed March 10, 2016. http://www.usccb.org/about/pro-life-activities/respect-life-program/killing-the-pain.cfm.

Dostoevsky, Fyodor. *The House of the Dead*. Translated by Julius Bramont. New York: Dover, 2004.

Dworkin, Ronald. *The Idiot*. Translated by David McDuff. Penguin: Amazon Digital Services, 2004.

———. *Sovereign Virtue: The Theory and Practice of Equality*. Cambridge, MA: Harvard University Press, 2000.

Eisenhower, General Dwight D. Accessed August 6, 2016. https://www.archives.gov/education/lessons/d-day-message/images/failure-message.gif.

Elliott, Carl. "Amputees by Choice." In *Better Than Well: American Medicine Meets the American Dream*, 208–36. New York: W. W. Norton, 2003.

Epictetus, *The Enchiridion, or Handbook* (Auckland: Floating Press, 2009).

Epicurus. "Letter to Menoeceus." Accessed September 17, 2014. http://www.epicurus.net/en/menoeceus.html.

Fink, Sheri. *Five Days at Memorial: Life and Death in a Storm-Ravaged Hospital*. New York: Broadway Books, 2016.

Fisher, Josie. "Re-Examining Death: Against a Higher Brain Criterion." *Journal of Medical Ethics* 25 (1999): 473–76.

Fisher, Leanne J. "The Suicide Trap: *Bouvia v. Superior Court* and the Right to Refuse Medical Treatment." *Loyola of Los Angeles Law Review*. 219/21 (1987).

Foster Wallace, David. "This Is Water." *Transcription of the 2005 Kenyon Commencement Address*. May 21, 2005. Accessed September 3, 2014. http://web.ics.purdue.edu/~drkelly/DFWKenyonAddress2005.pdf.

Frankfurt, Harry G. "Freedom of the Will and the Concept of a Person." *Journal of Philosophy* 68 no. 1 (January 1971): 5–20.

Freedman, Carol. "Aspirin for the Mind? Some Ethical Worries about Psychopharmacology." In *Enhancing Human Traits: Ethical and Social Implications*. Edited by Erik Parens. Washington, DC: Georgetown University Press, 1998.

Galvan, Astrid, and Justin Pritchard. "Feds Confiscate Lethal-Injection Drugs Obtained Overseas by Arizona and Texas." *U.S. News and World Report*. October 23, 2015. Accessed March 4, 2015. http://www.usnews.com/news/us/articles/2015/10/23/documents-arizona-tried-to-illegally-import-execution-drug.

Gawande, Atul. *Being Mortal: Medicine and What Matters in the End*. New York: Metropolitan Books, 2014.

Gorsuch, Neil. *The Future of Assisted Suicide and Euthanasia*. Princeton: Princeton University Press, 2009.

Greely, Henry T. "The Neuroscience Revolution, Ethics, and the Law." April 20, 2004. Accessed October 8, 2015. https://www.scu.edu/ethics/focusareas/bioethics/resources/the-neuroscience-revolution-ethics-and-the-law/.

Hadot, Pierre. *Philosophy as a Way of Life: Spiritual Exercises from Socrates to Foucault*. Malden, MA: Wiley-Blackwell, 1995.

Haliburton, Rachel. *Autonomy and the Situated Self: A Challenge to Bioethics*. Lanham, MD: Lexington Books, 2014.

Hardimon, Michael O. *Hegel's Social Philosophy: The Project of Reconciliation*. Cambridge: Cambridge University Press, 1994.

John Hardwig, "Going to Meet Death: The Art of Dying in the Early Part of the Twenty-First Century," *Hastings Center Report* 39, no. 4 (2009): 37–45.

———. ed., *Is There a Duty to Die? And Other Essays in Bioethics*. New York: Routledge, 2000.

Hari, Johann. *Chasing the Scream: The First and Last Days of the War on Drugs*. New York: Bloomsburg, 2015.

Harris, Sam. "The Self Is an Illusion." *Big Think*. September 16, 2014. Accessed March 5, 2015. https://www.youtube.com/watch?v=fajfkO_X0l0.

Harris, Sam, and Omer Aziz. Waking Up Podcast #32. March 12, 2016. Accessed July 30, 2017. https://www.samharris.org/podcast/item/the-best-podcast-ever.

Harris, Sam, and Rabbi David Wolpe. "Does God Exist?" April 24, 2012. Accessed May 28, 2016. https://www.youtube.com/watch?v=bN9nlAnkCUY.

Hays, Gregory. Introduction to Marcus Aurelius. In *Meditations*. Translated by Gregory Hays. New York: Modern Library, 2003.

Hensel, Wendy. "The Disabling Impact of Wrongful Birth and Wrongful Life Actions," *Harvard Civil Rights-Civil Liberties Law Review* 40 (2005): 141–95.

Herzberg, Abel. "The Holocaust: Crimes, Heroes, and Villains." Accessed January 4, 2015. http://www.auschwitz.dk/.

Hume, David. "My Own Life." April 18, 1776. Accessed July 29, 2015. http://isites.harvard.edu/fs/docs/icb.topic880131.files/My.Own.Life.by.David.Hume.pdf.

———. "Of Personal Identity." In *A Treatise of Human Nature*. Edited by P. H. Nidditch. Oxford: Clarendon Oxford, 1973.

Jabali-Nash, Naimah. "Husband Sacrifices Life for Pregnant Wife in Crash, Occupants of Oncoming Car on Drugs, Say Cops." *CBS News*. September 13, 2010. Accessed May 27, 2014. http://www.cbsnews.com/news/husband-sacrifices-life-for-pregnant-wife-in-crash-occupants-of-oncoming-car-on-drugs-say-cops/.

Jarvis Thompson, Judith. "A Defense of Abortion." *Philosophy and Public Affairs* 1, no. 1 (1971): 47–50.

Joung, J. Keith, and Jeffry D. Sander. "CRISPR-Cas9 Systems for Editing, Regulating, and Targeting Genomes." *Nature Biotechnology* 32 (2014): 347–55.

Junod, Tom. "The Falling Man." *Esquire Magazine*. September 2003. Accessed November 12, 2015. http://classic.esquire.com/the-falling-man/.

Kahane, Leo, and Stephen Shmanske. *The Oxford Handbook of Sports Economics. Vol. 1: The Economics of Sports*. Oxford: Oxford University Press, 2012.

Kant, Immanuel. *Groundwork for the Metaphysics of Morals*. Translated by Mary Gregor and Jens Timmermann. Cambridge: Cambridge University Press, 2012.

———. *Lectures on Ethics*. Edited and translated by Peter Heath, 144–49. Cambridge: Cambridge University Press, 1997.

———. *Metaphysics of Morals*. In *Practical Philosophy*. Translated by Mary Gregor. Cambridge: Cambridge University Press, 1996.

Kass, Leon. "Lingering Longer: Who Will Care?" *Washington Post*. September 29, 2005. Accessed May 23, 2016. http://www.washingtonpost.com/wpdyn/content/article/2005/09/28/AR2005092802119.html.

Kierkegaard, Søren. *Fear and Trembling*. Translated by Alastair Hannay. London: Penguin Classics, 1986.

———. *The Journals of Kierkegaard*. Translated by Alexander Dru. New York: Harper & Row, 1959.

Kramer, Peter. *Listening to Prozac: A Psychiatrist Explores Antidepressant Drugs and the Remaking of the Self*. Rev. ed. New York: Penguin Books, 1997.

Kymlicka, Will. *Liberalism, Community, and Culture*. Oxford: Clarendon, 1989.

Lachs, John. "When Abstract Moralizing Runs Amok." *Journal of Clinical Ethics* 5, no. 1 (1994): 10–13.

Lewis, C. S. "Men without Chests." In *The Abolition of Man*, 1–26. New York: HarperOne, 2015.

Lipuma, Samuel. "Continuous Sedation until Death as Physician Assisted Suicide/Euthanasia: A Conceptual Analysis." *Journal of Medicine and Philosophy* 38 (2013): 190–204.

Ludlow, Peter, Yujim Nagasawa, and Daniel Stoljar, eds., *There's Something about Mary: Essays on Phenomenal Consciousness and Frank Jackson's Knowledge Argument*. Cambridge: MIT University Press, 2004.

MacIntyre, Alasdair. "Does Applied Ethics Rest on a Mistake?" *Monist* 67, no. 4 (October 1984): 498–513.

Magnusson, Roger S. "The Devil's Choice: Re-Thinking Law, Ethics, and Symptom Relief in Palliative Care." *Journal of Law, Medicine, and Ethics* 34, no. 3 (Fall 2006): 559–69.

Mappes, Thomas. "Some Reflections on Advance Directives." *Newsletter on Philosophy and Medicine*, in *APA Newsletters* 98, no.1 (Fall 1998): 106–11.

Marquis, Don. "Why Abortion Is Immoral." *Journal of Philosophy* 86 (April 1989): 183–202.

McCauley, Robert. *Why Religion Is Natural and Science Is Not*. Oxford: Oxford University Press, 2013.

McColl Kennedy, Ian. "The Karen Quinlan Case: Problems and Proposals." *Journal of Medical Ethics* 2 (1976): 3–7.

McMahan, Jeff. "Killing Embryos for Stem Cell Research." *Metaphilosophy* 38, nos. 2–3 (2007): 178–83.

Michel, Vicki. "Suicide by Persons with Disabilities Disguised as the Refusal of Life-Sustaining Treatment." *HEC Forum* 7 (1995): 122–31.

Mohammed, Shan, and Elizabeth Peter. "Rituals, Death and the Moral Practice of Medical Futility." *Nursing Ethics* 2009 16, no. 3: 292–301.

Monk, Ray. *Ludwig Wittgenstein: The Duty of Genius*. New York: Penguin Books, 1991.

Montaigne, Michel de. "Of Custom," *Essays of Montaigne*. Vol. 1. Translated by Charles Cotton. Accessed August 15, 2016. http://oll.libertyfund.org/titles/montaigne-essays-of-montaigne-vol-1.

National Geographic Channel. "Funeral Strippers." *Taboo Video*. Accessed August 3, 2016. http://channel.nationalgeographic.com/taboo/videos/funeral-strippers/.

National World War II Museum. "D-Day Invasion." Accessed February 6, 2015. http://www.nationalww2museum.org/learn/education/for-students/ww2-history/d-day-june-6-1944.html.

New Orleans Pharmacy Museum. Accessed April 21, 2016.http://www.pharmacymuseum.org/about.

New York Task Force on Life and the Law. "When Death Is Sought—Assisted Suicide and Euthanasia in the Medical Context." Executive Summary, 1994. Accessed January 4, 2015. https://www.health.ny.gov/regulations/task_force/reports_publications/when_death_is_sought/preface.htm.

Nuremberg Code. "Trials of War Criminals before the Nuremberg Military Tribunals under Control Council Law No. 10." Vol. 2. Washington, DC: U.S. Government Printing Office. 1949.

O'Connor, Sandra Day. Concurring opinion in *Washington v. Glucksberg* and *Vacco v. Quill*. U.S. Supreme Court. 521 U.S. 702 (1997).

Olsen, Molly, Keith Swetz, and Paul Mueller. "Ethical Decision Making with End-of-Life Care: Palliative Sedation and Withholding or Withdrawing Life-Sustaining Treatments." *Mayo Clinic Proceedings* 85 (2010): 949–54.

O'Neill, Onora. *Autonomy and Trust in Bioethics*. Cambridge: Cambridge University Press, 2002.

Oregon Death with Dignity Act (1994). *Oregon Revised Statutes, 1996 Supplement*. 127.800–127.897.

Orentlicher, David. "The Supreme Court and Physician-Assisted Suicide: Rejecting Assisted Suicide but Embracing Euthanasia." *New England Journal of Medicine* 337 (1997): 1236–39.

Pagán, Victoria Emma, ed. *A Companion to Tacitus*. Malden, MA: Wiley-Blackwell, 2012.

PBS. "American Experience: D-Day." Accessed December 5, 2014. http://www.pbs.org/wgbh/amex/dday/peopleevents/p_rommel.html.

Pellegrino, Edmund. "The False Promise of Beneficent Killing." In *Regulating How We Die: The Ethical, Medical, and Legal Issues Surrounding Physician-Assisted Suicide*. Edited by Linda Emanuel, 71–91. Cambridge: Harvard University Press, 1998.

———. "Physician-Assisted Suicide and Euthanasia: Rebuttals of Rebuttals—The Moral Prohibition Remains." *Journal of Medicine and Philosophy* 26 (2001): 93–100.

Percy, Walker. *Love in the Ruins*. New York: Picador, 1999.

Pernick, Martin S. "Back from the Grave: Recurring Controversies over Defining and Diagnosing Death in History." In *Death: Beyond Whole-Brain Criteria*. Edited by Richard Zaner, 17–74. Boston: Kluwer Academic, 1988.

Philipps, Dave. "Suicide Rate among Veterans Has Risen Sharply since 2001." *New York Times*. July 7, 2016. Accessed August 13, 2016. http://www.nytimes.com/2016/07/08/us/suicide-rate-among-veterans-has-risen-sharply-since-2001.html?_r=0.

Plato, *Phaedo*. In *Plato: Complete Works*. Edited by John M. Cooper. Indianapolis: Hackett, 1997.

Portman, John. "Pneumonia, Friend of the Elderly." *Western Journal of Medicine* 173, no. 4 (October 2000): 277–78.

President's Council on Bioethics. "Human Cloning and Human Dignity: An Ethical Inquiry." In *Biomedical Ethics*. Edited by David DeGrazia et al., 516–17. New York: McGraw-Hill, 2011.

Quill, Timothy. "Death and Dignity: A Case of Individualized Decision Making." *New England Journal of Medicine* 324, no. 10 (March 1991): 691–94.

Rawls, John. "Outline of a Decision Procedure for Ethics." *Philosophical Review* 60, no. 2 (1951): 177–97.

Rehnquist, William H. Opinion of the court in *Washington v. Glucksberg*. U.S. Supreme Court. 521 U.S. 702 (1997).

Rhodes, Rosamond. "Understanding the Trusted Doctor and Constructing a Theory of Bioethics." *Theoretical Medicine* 22 (2001): 493–504.

Rie, Michael. "Practicing Medicine, Fiduciary Trust Privacy, and Public Moral Interloping after '*Cruzan*.'" *Journal of Medicine and Philosophy* 17, no. 6 (1992): 647–64.

Robinson, Howard. "Dennett on the Knowledge Argument." *Analysis* 53, no.3 (July 1993): 174–77.

Sacks, Oliver. "My Own Life." *New York Times*. February 19, 2015. Accessed October 2, 2015. http://www.nytimes.com/2015/02/19/opinion/oliver-sacks-on-learning-he-has-terminal-cancer.html?_r=0.

Salter, Jim. "Missouri Governor Halts First U.S. Execution by Propofol." *Washington Post*. October 11, 2013. Accessed November 7, 2015. https://www.washingtonpost.com/politics/missouri-gov-halts-1st-us-execution-by-propofol/2013/10/11/559e6af6–32d9–11e3–8627-c5d7de0a046b_story.html.

Scheffler, Samuel. *Death and the Afterlife*. New York: Oxford University Press, 2013.

Schwartz, Barry. *The Paradox of Choice: Why Less is More*. Rev. ed. New York: HarperCollins, 2016.

Scott, Mike. "For Steve Gleason and Family, New Documentary Is 'As Real as It Can Get.'" July 22, 2016. Accessed July 23, 2016. http://www.nola.com/movies/index.ssf/2016/07/steve_gleason_documentary_mich.html.

Seneca, Lucius Annaeus. *Moral Epistles*. Translated by Richard M. Gummere. *Loeb Classical Library* 75. Cambridge: Harvard University Press, 1917.

Sextus Empiricus. *Outlines of Skepticism*. Edited by Julia Annas and Jonathan Barnes. Cambridge: Cambridge University Press, 2000.

Simerman, John, and Ramon Antonio Vargas. "'Penile Plethysmograph' Test to Gauge Arousal Part of Darren Sharper's Strict Post-prison Deal." *New Orleans Advocate*. April 14, 2015. Accessed June 5, 2016. http://www.theadvocate.com/new_orleans/news/article_a0ccb184–5acd-5508-bfec-6982605b5fac.html.

Singer, Peter. "The Singer Solution to World Poverty." *New York Times*. September 5, 1999.

Slotnik, Daniel E. "Brittany Maynard, 'Death with Dignity Ally, Dies at 29." *New York Times*. November 3, 2014.

Steadman, Ian. "U.S. Prisons, Foiled by an EU Boycott, Are Turning to Untested Drugs in Executions." January 14, 2014. Accessed March 25, 2015. http://www.newstatesman.com/future-proof/2014/01/us-prisons-foiled-eu-boycott-are-turning-untested-drugs-executions.

Sumner, Wayne. "And When I Die: The Pro-Life Case for Assisted Suicide." October 15, 2014. Accessed December 4, 2015. http://thewalrus.ca/and-when-i-die/.

Sykes, Nigel, and Andrew Thorns. "The Use of Opioids and Sedatives at the End of Life." *Lancet Oncology* 1 (2003): 312–18.

Szpir, Michael. "An Interview with Carl Elliott." Accessed February 15, 2015. http://www.americanscientist.org/bookshelf/pub/carl-elliott.

Thornton, K. and C. B. Phillips. "Performing the Good Death: The Medieval Ars Moriendi and Contemporary Doctors." *Medical Humanities* 35, no. 2 (2009): 94–97.

Tolstoy, Leo. *The Death of Ivan Ilyich*. Translated by Lynn Solotaroff. New York: Bantam Dell, 1981.

Truog, Robert, and Franklin Miller. "The Dead Donor Rule and Organ Transplantation," *New England Journal of Medicine* 359 (2008): 674–675.

Unger, Peter. *Living High and Letting Die: Our Illusion of Innocence*. New York: Oxford University Press, 1996.

Uniform Law Commission. "The Uniform Determination of Death Act." Accessed October 20, 2015, http://www.uniformlaws.org/shared/docs/determination%20of%20death/udda80.pdf.

Vacco v. Quill, 521 U.S. 793 (1997).

Veatch, Robert. "The Death of Whole-brain Death: The Plague of the Disaggregators, Somaticists, and Mentalists." *Journal of Medicine and Philosophy* 30, no. 4 (2005): 353–78.

———. "Donating Hearts after Cardiac Death—Reversing the Irreversible." *New England Journal of Medicine* 359 (2008): 672–73.

Veatch, Robert, and Lainie Ross. *Defining Death: The Case for Choice*. Washington, DC: Georgetown University Press, 2016.

Velleman, J. David. "Against the Right to Die." *Journal of Medicine and Philosophy* 17 (1992): 665–81.

Verhagen, Edward, and Pieter J. J. Sauer. "The Groningen Protocol—Euthanasia in Severely Ill Newborns." *New England Journal of Medicine* 352, no. 10 (2005): 959–62.

Warren, Mary Anne. "On the Moral and Legal Status of Abortion." *Monist* 57 no.1 (January 1973): 43–61.

White, Tracie. "Most Physicians Would Forgo Aggressive Treatment for Themselves at the End of Life, Study Finds." *Stanford Medicine News Center*. May 28, 2014. Accessed July 16, 2016. https://med.stanford.edu/news/all-news/2014/05/most-physicians-would-forgo-aggressive-treatment-for-themselves-.html.

Whole Woman's Health v. Hellerstedt. U.S. Supreme Court. Decided June 27, 2016. Accessed August 15, 2016. https://www.supremecourt.gov/opinions/15pdf/15–274_p8k0.pdf.

Wicclair, Mark. *Ethics and the Elderly*. Oxford: Oxford University Press, 1993.

Wikler, Daniel. "What Has Bioethics to Offer Health Policy?" *Millbank Quarterly* 69, no. 2 (1991): 233–51.

Winston, Kenneth I. "On Treating Like Cases Alike." *California Law Review*. 62/1 (1974).

Wittgenstein, Ludwig. *Lecture on Ethics*. November 1929. Accessed May 30, 2015. http://sackett.net/WittgensteinEthics.pdf.

Yeo, Michael. "Primum Non Nocere: The Ethics of Teaching Medical Ethics," *Teaching Philosophy* 12, no. 1 (March 1989): 23–34.

Index

www.ingramcontent.com/pod-product-compliance
Ingram Content Group UK Ltd.
Pitfield, Milton Keynes, MK11 3LW, UK
UKHW041626031026
15587UKWH00001B/89

9 780739 199213